D1478711

Neurofibromatosis

A Handbook for Patients, Families, and Health Care Professionals

Second Edition

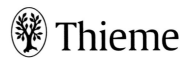 Thieme

Key to Cover Images

Top: Angiogram showing moya-moya phenomenon due to carotid artery occlusion.

Middle: Fluorescence in situ hybridization image showing *NF1* gene labeled on each copy of chromosome 17. (Photo courtesy of Dr. Andrew Carroll, University of Alabama at Birmingham, with permission.)

Bottom: Fluorescence staining of culture Schwann cells from a neurofibroma. (Photo courtesy of Dr. Ludwine Messiaen, University of Alabama at Birmingham, and Ophelia Maertens, University Hospital, Gent, Belgium, with permission.)

Neurofibromatosis

A Handbook for Patients, Families, and Health Care Professionals

Second Edition

Bruce R. Korf, M.D., Ph.D.
Wayne H. and Sara Crews Finley Professor
    of Medical Genetics
Chair, Department of Genetics
University of Alabama at Birmingham

Allan E. Rubenstein, M.D.
Clinical Associate Professor of Neurology
Mount Sinai School of Medicine
CEO, NexGenix Pharmaceuticals, LLC
New York, New York

Thieme Medical Publishers
New York • Stuttgart

Thieme New York
333 Seventh Avenue
New York, NY 10001

Senior Editor: Timothy Y. Hiscock
Assistant Editor: Birgitta Brandenburg
Director, Production and Manufacturing: Anne Vinnicombe
Senior Production Editor: David R. Stewart
Marketing Director: Phyllis Gold
Director of Sales: Ross Lumpkin
Chief Financial Officer: Peter van Woerden
President: Brian D. Scanlan
Compositor: Thomson Press (India) Limited
Printer: The Maple-Vail Book Manufacturing Group

Library of Congress Cataloging in Publication Data is available from the publisher

Important note: Medical knowledge is ever-changing. As new research and clinical
experience broaden our knowledge, changes in treatment and drug therapy may be
required. The authors and editors of the material herein have consulted sources believed
to be reliable in their efforts to provide information that is complete and in accord with
the standards accepted at the time of publication. However, in view of the possibility of
human error by the authors, editors, or publisher of the work herein, or changes in medical
knowledge, neither the authors, editors, or publisher, nor any other party who has been
involved in the preparation of this work, warrants that the information contained herein is
in every respect accurate or complete, and they are not responsible for any errors or
omissions or for the results obtained from use of such information. Readers are encouraged
to confirm the information contained herein with other sources. For example, readers are
advised to check the product information sheet included in the package of each drug
they plan to administer to be certain that the information contained in this publication
is accurate and that changes have not been made in the recommended dose or in the
contraindications for administration. This recommendation is of particular importance
in connection with new or infrequently used drugs.

Some of the product names, patents, and registered designs referred to in this book are in
fact registered trademarks or proprietary names even though specific reference to this fact
is not always made in the text. Therefore, the appearance of a name without designation as
proprietary is not to be construed as a representation by the publisher that it is in the
public domain.

Printed in the United States of America

5 4 3 2 1

TNY ISBN 1-58890-301-X
GTV ISBN 3-13-655102-2

Dedicated to all those who have neurofibromatosis and their families

Contents

Preface

The first edition of this book was published in 1990. It was written during an exciting time in the neurofibromatosis community: the genes for NF1 and NF2 had just been mapped and the NIH recently had held its consensus conference on diagnosis and management of neurofibromatosis. In fact, neurofibromatosis research was then just turning a corner. It had been about 100 years since von Recklinghausen's seminal work that defined the disorder. Many refinements had been made in clinical care, especially in surgery and imaging, but the 1990 approach to diagnosis and management would, in many ways, have been familiar to a 19th century physician such as von Recklinghausen. The ensuing 15 years, however, have seen dramatic changes. These have been a source of great hope for those who must deal with neurofibromatosis, whether as a patient, a family member, or a physician.

Many of the changes are the result of general advances in medicine, not specific to neurofibromatosis. The use of magnetic resonance imaging (MRI) is a dramatic example of a technology that was just emerging when the first edition of this book was published but which is now routine. It is hard to imagine taking care of a person with NF1 or NF2 without the benefit of MRI to precisely define the extent and rate of growth of major tumors. Approaches to management have also improved, including better surgical techniques and new forms of chemotherapy. For example, substitution of watchful waiting or chemotherapy for radiation therapy has vastly improved the quality of care for children with NF1 and optic glioma.

Other advances — the ones that have generated the most excitement — are those that have revealed the basic mechanisms by which the neurofibromatoses exert their effects on the body. These advances flow from the ability to study the neurofibromatosis genes, the proteins encoded by those genes, and the way these proteins behave in cells and in animal models. Although much remains to be learned about the disorders, the cellular pathways that are disturbed in individuals with neurofibromatosis are rapidly coming into focus. This has spawned genetic tests and is beginning to generate insights that may lead to new treatments. Families now have a realistic expectation that an individual who has NF might be eligible to participate in a clinical trial, a notion that was unheard of in 1990.

As rapidly as advances are being made, they can never happen fast enough for those who are affected by neurofibromatosis. In spite of the power of modern medical research, there is still a significant lag between discovery of a gene or cellular mechanism and the ability to use this information for treatment. The more that is learned, the greater the respect that scientists have for the complexity of any biological system. We cannot yet say that light is visible at the end of the neurofibromatosis tunnel, but at least we are now traveling through the tunnel on a high-speed train rather than walking.

The first edition of this book was written originally for patients, families, and health care providers. Since it was published, several books have been written for professionals, but no others for patients and families. This new edition has been completely rewritten, and is specifically targeted towards this latter audience. It was written in the spirit that having a better understanding of neurofibromatosis is the first step towards taking charge and dealing with it. We are grateful to many colleagues who have provided advice, and to many patients and families who have shared their personal stories.

We thank the employees, directors, and members of the National Neurofibromatosis Foundation, Inc., Peter W.R. Bellermann, president; Ann MacDonald, writer; Jane Novak Pugh, editor and project manager, whose efforts made this book possible.

When the first edition was written we expressed the hope in the preface that our foresight would prove to be myopic. It was: research has revealed insights we could not have imagined at the time. It is certain that the next 15 years will produce even more dramatic insights and surprises. No one can say when these will result in new treatments, but the prospects for a person diagnosed today with neurofibromatosis have never been brighter.

Bruce R. Korf, M.D., Ph.D.
Allan E. Rubenstein, M.D.

1

Introduction and History

Neurofibromatosis* is the umbrella term for three distinct genetic disorders that share a hallmark manifestation—*tumor* growth in the tissues that surround nerves. Most tumors are *benign*, although occasionally they can become *malignant*. Neurofibromatosis may also cause additional complications. None of these disorders is the so-called Elephant Man's disease, a persistent misconception that sometimes alarms people who have just received a diagnosis themselves or for a child. The life of Joseph Merrick dramatized in a movie and in a play, both titled *The Elephant Man,* helped to focus public attention on these disorders.

It is important to note at the outset that the neurofibromatoses are classified not as diseases but as disorders. Although these two words are sometimes used interchangeably, they do have quite distinct medical connotations. A person with a disease, from whatever cause, feels ill, whereas a person with a disorder may or may not experience medical problems. People contract an illness; they are born with a disorder and it is part of their basic makeup. Many people diagnosed with neurofibromatosis experience few medical complications arising from the disorder; some are so mildly affected that they may never even receive a diagnosis.

Though they are often referred to as "rare," the neurofibromatoses are surprisingly common. They are more prevalent than cystic fibrosis, Duchenne muscular dystrophy, Huntington's disease, and Tay-Sachs disease combined (Table **1–1**). Neurofibromatosis 1 (NF1) is by far

---

*Italicized terms are defined in the glossary.

Table 1–1   Prevalence of Genetic Disorders

Disorder	Estimated Birth Incidence
Neurofibromatosis 1	1 in 3,000 to 4,000
Neurofibromatosis 2	1 in 40,000
Schwannomatosis	Not yet documented but appears to be the same as NF2
Cystic fibrosis	1 in 2,000 (in white people) 1 in 90,000 (nonwhite people)
Duchenne muscular dystrophy	1 in 3,500 males (rarely affects females)
Huntington's disease	1 in 20,000
Tay-Sachs disease	1 in 2,500 (in Ashkenazi Jews) 1 in 250,000 (rest of population)

the most common form, occurring in 10 times more people than neurofibromatosis 2 (NF2).[1] A third type of neurofibromatosis, *schwannomatosis*, appears to occur as often as NF2 (see Chapter 12).

Neurofibromatosis occurs without regard to sex, race, or ethnic origin. Although methods of determining incidence and prevalence vary, the National Institutes of Health (NIH) has estimated that more than 100,000 Americans have neurofibromatosis.[2] About half of the cases of NF1 and NF2 are inherited or *familial* in nature; the other half are *sporadic* cases that develop because of a spontaneous change in a *gene*. This is not the case in schwannomatosis. These three disorders—NF1, NF2, and schwannomatosis—can present in almost any family, and any physician might face the challenge of diagnosing and treating persons with one of them.

◆ Growing Insight into Neurofibromatosis

Key events in the history of neurofibromatosis are detailed in Table **1–2**. Case reports of people who apparently had neurofibromatosis began to appear in the late 18th century in various languages. Reports then continued to accumulate into the 19th and 20th centuries. Throughout that time, what are now known as NF1, NF2, and schwannomatosis were not seen as separate disorders, or even classified as *syndromes*. Instead, individual manifestations were documented, laying the groundwork for the genetic insights that took place starting in the late 20th century.

What is probably the first illustration of someone with NF1 dates back to the 13th century. It is credited to an Austrian monk known for his

Table 1–2   Significant Milestones in Neurofibromatosis

Date	Milestone	Reference
13th century	The first known drawing is made of a man who may have had NF1.	3 (p. 3)
1785	Mark Akenside, a British physician, publishes the first English-language description of someone with NF1 manifestations.	4
1793	A case report is published about Johann Gottfried Rheinhard, who had multiple wart-like growths covering his skin, a large head, and areas of skin discoloration. This is the most detailed early account of someone with NF1.	5
1822	In what is probably the first description of NF2, Scottish physician J. H. Wishart describes a patient with multiple intracranial meningiomas and cranial tumors, including acoustic neuromas.	7
1830	Schwann identifies a myelin sheath cell that is later recognized as the most common type of cell in NF tumors.	3 (p. 5)
1882	Friedrich Daniel von Recklinghausen, a pathologist in Strassburg, publishes a landmark monograph about the disorder that would later bear his name. He coins the term *neurofibroma* after observing that NF tumors were composed of nerve cells and fibrous supportive tissue.	18
1880s to 1970s	Case reports are published that describe families with multiple members affected by NF1 and NF2. Physicians and researchers identify and begin to better understand the many types of cells involved and the clinical pathology of these disorders.	
1978	The National Neurofibromatosis Foundation is founded by Lynn Courtemanche, R.N., Allan Rubenstein, M.D., and Joel Hirschtritt, Esq.	
1979	The NF Foundation establishes the first comprehensive NF clinic. (Others will follow.)	
1983	The NF Foundation launches the first national research program on neurofibromatosis in the world.	
1987	The National Institutes of Health hosts a landmark consensus development conference that creates the nomenclature "NF1" and "NF2," establishes diagnostic criteria for both disorders, and provides guidelines for treatment.	1,19–22
	The NNFF International Consortium for the Molecular Biology of NF1 and NF2 is established, in which researchers agree to share molecular and clinical data. The consortium has grown from 32 scientists in 1987 to more than 300 today, and has helped speed the progress of research into NF.	
	Scientists identify genetic markers for NF1 on chromosome 17 and for NF2 on chromosome 22. This significantly narrows the search for the causative genes.	

(Continued)

Table 1–2   (Continued)

Date	Milestone	Reference
1988	The first diagnostic DNA, prenatal, and presymptomatic testing for familial cases of NF1 is developed.	
1990	Two teams working independently identify the NF1 gene and describe its protein.	2,23–25
	The National Institutes of Health sponsors a clinical conference to review and update guidelines for the diagnosis and management of NF1 and NF2.	
1992	The NF Foundation forms the International Neurofibromatosis Association in Luxembourg.	
1993	Scientists identify the NF2 gene and describe its protein product.	26,27
	The NF Foundation establishes an international network of clinics to improve diagnosis and treatment of people with NF1 and NF2.	
1994	The first multicenter clinical trials are launched to test new therapies for people with NF.	
1995	Direct gene testing becomes available for NF1 and NF2. (The tests are available only in the research setting, for reasons discussed in Chapter 2.)	
1997	The NF Foundation Clinical Care Advisory Board leads a worldwide effort to provide an updated consensus about diagnostic and management criteria for NF1 and NF2.	11
1990 to present	Researchers advance knowledge of how the NF1 and NF2 gene mutations contribute to these disorders' manifestations, including tumor formation and cognitive difficulties.	28
	Researchers establish that schwannomatosis is genetically distinct from NF2 and consensus builds that it represents a third form of neurofibromatosis.	

illustrations of amphibians, but may have been done by someone else.[3(p3)] Another 500 years would pass before, in 1785, the first English-language description of the disorder was published.[4] In 1793, W. G. von Tilesius wrote about a patient his professor, Christian Friedrich Ludwig, referred to as the "wart man."[5] The patient, Johann Gottfried Rheinhard (Fig. **1–1**), had multiple fibrous tumors visible on his skin that resemble dermal neurofibromas.

The man who is most responsible for synthesizing these various observations and case reports was a German professor of pathology, Friedrich Daniel von Recklinghausen (Fig. **1–2**), who in 1882 coined the term *neurofibroma* (from "neuro" for nerve and "fibroma" for fibrous tissue). In his landmark monograph, *On Multiple Fibromas of the Skin and Their Relationship to Multiple Neuromas*, von Recklinghausen also was the first to realize that tumors common in this disorder arose from cells that help to form the protective myelin sheath around nerves. In recognition of his

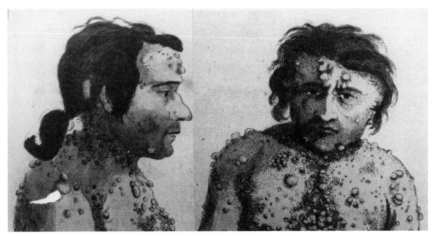

Figure 1–1   Detail of drawings of Johann Gottfried Rheinhard, who was called Wart Man by Professor Christian Friedrich Ludwig. Original drawings are in color in the 1793 report by Tilesius, a student of Ludwig's.

contributions, what is now known as NF1 was first called "von Recklinghausen's disease." As clues continued to accumulate into the 20th century, additional manifestations were associated with the disorder, such as *café-au-lait spots*, *Lisch nodules*, skeletal abnormalities, and rare malignancies.

The first description of NF2 is credited in the early 1800s to J. H. Wishart, a Scottish physician who published a case report about one

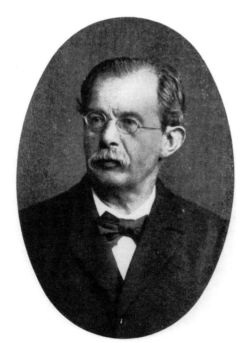

Figure 1–2 Friedrich Daniel von Recklinghausen (1833–1910, Professor of Pathology, Strassburg), around the time that he wrote his monograph, *On Multiple Fibromas of the Skin and Their Relationship to Multiple Neuromas.* (Courtesy of the National Library of Medicine.)

of his patients. The young man became deaf by the time he was 19 and died during surgery 2 years later. An autopsy revealed multiple tumors at the base and in the lining of his skull, as well as tumors along the *cranial* nerves that are now recognized as an NF2 hallmark.[6,7] More than a century later, W. J. Gardner and C. H. Frazier published a report about five generations of a family affected by what appears to be NF2; 38 members of the family were deaf in both ears.[8] This more fully characterized the disorder and showed that it is hereditary.

In the meantime, two German physicians proposed that there might in fact be two distinct types of neurofibromatosis, which they called "central" and "peripheral" neurofibromatosis. They correctly observed that people with central neurofibromatosis do not usually have café-au-lait spots and skin tumors, but do tend to have nerve tumors that impair hearing.[9] Although many researchers continued to regard the two disorders as one, gradually it became clear that they are clinically distinct. Eldridge[10] coined the term *bilateral acoustic neurofibromatosis* in 1981 in a report that identified such tumors as a hallmark sign of the central type of the disorder.

Participants in the NIH consensus conference, held in 1987, created a common nomenclature for the two most common types of neurofibromatosis.[1] Von Recklinghausen's disease, also known as peripheral neurofibromatosis, was designated NF1. Central neurofibromatosis, also known as bilateral acoustic neurofibromatosis, was designated NF2. The NIH panel established diagnostic criteria and guidelines for management. Both the diagnostic criteria and management guidelines have been reviewed and updated, once in 1990,[2] and again in 1997.[11] Diagnostic criteria have been proposed for schwannomatosis (see Chapter 12), although further research is necessary before consensus is possible.

◆ The Elephant Man

Joseph Merrick, the unfortunate individual who would become known as the "Elephant Man," was born in Leicester, England, in 1862. By the time he was 18 months old, abnormal growths appeared on his face. As he grew older, huge cauliflower-like masses made of thickened skin covered his head and body. His right arm became grotesquely swollen.[12] After his mother died, Merrick joined a series of freak shows. One imaginative promoter dubbed him the "Elephant Man" and claimed that Merrick's deformities developed after his mother was trampled by an elephant while pregnant with him.

Sir Frederick Treves, a distinguished London surgeon who had provided medical advice and services to Queen Victoria and other members of the Royal Family, first met Merrick by chance and later befriended him. Treves presented Merrick's case at a medical society meeting, then gradually introduced the young man to Victorian society, where he became something of a celebrity. Sadly, Merrick's medical condition worsened, and he died when he was 28 years old. Treves subsequently published a brief case report and later a book about Merrick's life.[13,14]

The story probably would have ended there, but interest revived in the 1970s after physical and cultural anthropologist Ashley Montagu published a book about Merrick's life that emphasized his dignity and humanity.[15] Montagu's work generated so much interest that both a play and a movie were independently developed at approximately the same time.[16]

Scientists had long wondered what caused Merrick's deformities. In 1909 the British dermatologist F. Parkes Weber published a paper speculating that Merrick may have had an "incomplete" type of neurofibromatosis, then known as von Recklinghausen's disease.[17] Although Merrick never developed café-au-lait spots, by then recognized as a common feature of NF1, Parkes Weber's theory became widely accepted. This actually proved to be a blessing for neurofibromatosis research. The book and the movie about the Elephant Man raised awareness of neurofibromatosis, and donations, just as improved genetic technology was narrowing the search for the causative genes.

It turns out, however, that Merrick probably did not have neurofibromatosis. Two Canadian geneticists published a report in 1986 claiming that Merrick might have had Proteus syndrome, a rare and then only recently identified disorder that involves multiple types of malformations.[12] The basic difference is that neurofibromatosis is expressed in nerve tissue, whereas Proteus syndrome results in abnormal growth of bone, skin, and other soft tissues.[16] Although the debate about exactly what disorder Merrick endured continues, the consensus now is that whatever it was, it was not neurofibromatosis.

◆ Information and Support

This book is written for patients, families, and physicians. It includes information about the manifestations of neurofibromatosis, the usual progression of these disorders, what options exist for treatment, and where to find support. Also included are the personal stories and perspectives of people with neurofibromatosis and their families.

There is currently no way to prevent or cure neurofibromatosis; however, consensus does exist about how to monitor and manage complications. The responsible genes for both NF1 and NF2 have been identified, and scientists are now unraveling the sequence of biological events that lead to development of tumors and other manifestations. This will also help to identify new targets for therapy. The mechanism responsible for schwannomatosis had not yet been found at the time this book went to press, but the research continues.

Genetic tests for both NF1 and NF2 are used in research studies but are just becoming available on a clinical basis. For the most part they have little to offer in terms of guiding or improving therapy. Clinical criteria and guidelines for diagnosis and management have been established for NF1 and NF2, and proposed for schwannomatosis. Because tumors in neurofibromatosis are usually slow growing and rarely turn malignant, the best strategy is often one of "watchful waiting." The tendency in the past to conduct multiple diagnostic tests and intervene early with surgery and other types of therapy has given way to a more conservative approach. Fortunately, many people with neurofibromatosis experience only mild to moderate manifestations.

References

1. National Institutes of Health. NIH. Neurofibromatosis Consensus Development Conference. Neurofibromatosis Conference Statement. Arch Neurol 1988;45:575–578
2. National Institutes of Health Conference. Neurofibromatosis 1 (Recklinghausen disease) and neurofibromatosis 2 (bilateral acoustic neurofibromatosis): an update. Ann Intern Med 1990;113:39–52
3. Mulvihill JJ. Introduction and History. In: Rubenstein AE, Korf BR, eds. Neurofibromatosis: A Handbook for Patients, Families, and Health-Care Professionals. New York: Thieme Medical Publishers; 1990
4. Akenside M. Observations on cancers. Med Trans Coll Physicians London 1785;1:64–92
5. von Tilesius WG. Historia Pathologica Singularis Cutis Turpitudinis. J Godofredi Rheinhardi Viri 50 Annorum. Leipzig: S.L. Crusius; 1793
6. Friedman JM, Gutmann DH, MacCollin M, Riccardi VM, eds. Neurofibromatosis: Phenotype, Natural History, and Pathogenesis. 3rd ed. Baltimore: Johns Hopkins University Press; 1999:299
7. Wishart JH. Case of tumours in the skull, dura matter, and brain. Edinburgh Med Surg J 1822;18:393–397
8. Gardner WJ, Frazier CH. Bilateral acoustic neurofibromatosis: a clinical study and field survey of a family of five generations with bilateral deafness in thirty-eight members. Arch Neurol Psychiatry 1930;23:266–302
9. Henneberg K, Koch M. Ueber "centrale" neurofibromatose und die Geschwulste des Klein-hirnbruckenwinkels (acusticusneurome). Arch Psy Nervenkr 1903;36:251–304. Cited by: Friedman JM, Gutmann DH, MacCollin M, Riccardi VM, eds. Neurofibromatosis: Phenotype, Natural History, and Pathogenesis. 3rd ed. Baltimore: Johns Hopkins University Press; 1999:299
10. Eldridge R. Central neurofibromatosis with bilateral acoustic neuroma. Adv Neurol 1981;29:57–65
11. Gutmann DH, Aylsworth A, Carey JC, et al. The diagnostic evaluation and multidisciplinary management of neurofibromatosis 1 and neurofibromatosis 2. JAMA 1997;278:51–57
12. Tibbles JAR, Cohen MM Jr. The Proteus syndrome: the Elephant Man diagnosed. Br Med J (Clin Res Ed) 1986;293:683–685
13. Treves F. A case of congenital deformity. Trans Pathol Soc London 1885;36:494–498
14. Treves F. The Elephant Man and Other Reminiscences. London: Cassell; 1923

15. Montagu A. The Elephant Man: A Study in Human Dignity. London: Outerbridge & Dienstfrey; 1971
16. Aronson J. Protean elephants. BMJ 1998;316:89
17. Weber FP. Cutaneous pigmentations as an incomplete form of Recklinghausen's disease, with remarks on the classification of incomplete and anomalous forms of Recklinghausen's disease. Br J Dermatol 1909;21:49–53
18. von Recklinghausen FD. Ueber die Multiplen Fibrome der Haut und ihre Beziehung zu den Multiplen Neuromen. Berlin: Hirschwald; 1882
19. Barker D, Wright E, Nguyen L, et al. Gene for von Recklinghausen neurofibromatosis is in the pericentromeric region of chromosome 17. Science 1987;236:1100–1102
20. Seizinger BR, Rouleau GA, Ozelius LJ, et al. Genetic linkage of von Recklinghausen neurofibromatosis to the nerve growth factor receptor gene. Cell 1987;49:589–594
21. Seizinger BR, Martuza RL, Gusella JF. Loss of genes on chromosome 22 in tumorigenesis of human acoustic neuroma. Nature 1986;322:644–647
22. Seizinger BR, Rouleau G, Ozelius LJ, et al. Common pathogenetic mechanism for three tumor types in bilateral acoustic neurofibromatosis. Science 1987;236:317–319
23. Wallace MR, Marchuk DA, Andersen LB, et al. Type 1 neurofibromatosis gene: identification of a large transcript disrupted in three NF1 patients. Science 1990;249:181–186
24. Cawthon RM, Weiss M, Xu G, et al. A major segment of the neurofibromatosis type 1 gene: cDNA sequence, genomic structure, and point mutations. Cell 1990;62:193–201
25. Viskochil D, Buchberg AM, Xu G, et al. Deletions and a translocation interrupt a cloned gene at the neurofibromatosis type 1 locus. Cell 1990;62:187–192
26. Trofatter JA, MacCollin MM, Rutter JL, et al. A novel moesin-, ezrin-, radixin-like gene is a candidate for the neurofibromatosis 2 tumor suppressor. Cell 1993;72:791–800
27. Rouleau GA, Merel P, Lutchman M, et al. Alteration in a new gene encoding a putative membrane-organizing protein causes neurofibromatosis type 2. Nature 1993;363:515–521
28. MacCollin M, Willett C, Heinrich B, et al. Familial schwannomatosis: exclusion of the NF2 locus as the germline event. Neurology 2003;60:1968–1974

2

The Many Faces of Neurofibromatosis

The diagnosis of neurofibromatosis is based on clinical criteria established mainly through a detailed medical history and physical examination. Although other varieties of neurofibromatosis may exist, genes have been found, and diagnostic criteria established through consensus committees, for only two: neurofibromatosis 1 (NF1) and neurofibromatosis 2 (NF2). Criteria have been proposed for a third type of neurofibromatosis, schwannomatosis, as the search for its cause continues.

The current criteria to diagnose NF1 and NF2 were issued in 1997 by the National Neurofibromatosis Foundation Clinical Care Advisory Board.[1] The board not only reviewed and updated diagnostic criteria and management guidelines issued originally in 1987, and updated in 1990, by the National Institutes of Health,[2,3] but also conducted its own independent review of relevant research studies.

In most cases, the criteria detailed in Chapters 5, 10, and 12 can be used to establish or rule out a diagnosis of neurofibromatosis. Because many features of these disorders are age dependent, however, diagnosis may take several years, especially if there is no family medical history of neurofibromatosis. Although this may frustrate patients and their families, at this point there are few alternatives to a strategy of watchful waiting. No laboratory test establishes the diagnosis, although sometimes tissue biopsies or radiological films, such as magnetic resonance imaging (*MRI*) scans and x-rays, provide additional information to help confirm one. Even though the genes for both NF1 and NF2 have been identified and clinical genetic testing is available, it is not appropriate for everyone and in most cases does not influence management of the disorders (see Chapter 4). Nor is there a reliable blood test: the NF1 and NF2 proteins both function inside cells and therefore cannot be measured in the same way as blood sugar, cholesterol, and other biological products that circulate in the bloodstream. The responsible mechanism for schwannomatosis has not yet been identified and no genetic test exists.

Although it is human nature to want to know something definitive, it is important to remember that in most cases early diagnosis of neurofibromatosis does not have an effect on management of these disorders. The most productive strategy, for physicians and patients alike, is to adopt an attitude of informed vigilance. (This chapter and the ones that follow provide information to facilitate doing just that.)

◆ Common Features of Neurofibromatosis

The neurofibromatoses are primarily evident in cells and connective tissue in the nervous system, but they are otherwise distinct. Given their significantly different clinical manifestations, it is somewhat surprising to think that NF1 and NF2 were once thought of as a single entity. Schwannomatosis is somewhat harder to distinguish from NF2 because the two disorders share a hallmark tumor type. Table **2–1** presents a quick summary of the differences between NF1, NF2, and schwannomatosis.

Tumors in neurofibromatosis grow from cells and tissues that play essential roles in the functioning of the nervous system (Fig. **2–1**). NF1 mainly affects nerve sheath cells in the *peripheral nervous system*. Its hallmark features include multiple café-au-lait spots and neurofibromas. The signature manifestation in NF2, which mostly is revealed in the central nervous system, is bilateral *schwannomas* that grow on the vestibular nerve, which connects the inner ear to the brain. Schwannomatosis was once considered a subtype of NF2 because it also causes multiple schwannomas to grow. In schwannomatosis, however, the tumors grow anywhere except on the vestibular nerve. Although it is possible that other types of neurofibromatosis exist, this is difficult to determine with certainty because these disorders vary widely in symptoms and severity.

The cells that compose the nervous system are unique in that they form large networks and interdependent circuits that snake beneath the skin to every point in the body. *Neurons*, individual nerve cells in the brain

Table 2–1   Distinguishing Features of NF1, NF2, and Schwannomatosis

Typical Characteristic	NF1	NF2	Schwannomatosis
Gene location	Chromosome 17	Chromosome 22	Unknown but likely chromosome 22
Onset of manifestations	Early childhood	Early adulthood	Early adulthood
First manifestations	Café-au-lait spots	Hearing and/or balance problems	Pain
Eye manifestations	Lisch nodules	Posterior subcapsular cataracts	None
Common developmental aspects	Large head Short stature Learning disabilities	None	None
Most common tumors	Neurofibromas Optic gliomas	Schwannomas (especially vestibular) Meningiomas	Schwannomas (any except vestibular)

and spinal cord, rely on a vast network of connections with other nerve cells to help people sense, move, and think. Nerve cells are connected by *axons,* which transmit electrical impulses much like wires in a house.

In neurofibromatosis, tumors primarily develop in support cells that surround nerve cells and help them to function. The cells most often involved are those that help to form protective insulation around axons known as the *myelin* sheath. In the brain and spinal cord, oligodendrocytes help to form myelin; in the peripheral nervous system *Schwann cells* perform this role. Connective tissue in the nervous system contains fibroblasts and meningeal cells. Astrocytes clean up excess transmitters and ions (which help neurons to communicate) and provide glucose to fuel neuronal activity. All of these cells have been found in various types of tumors caused by neurofibromatosis.

◆ Distinguishing Neurofibromatosis 1 from Neurofibromatosis 2

Although the consensus criteria and the discovery of two separate genes make it clear that NF1 and NF2 are two distinct disorders, the two are still sometimes confused at diagnosis. Most often, this occurs when a person

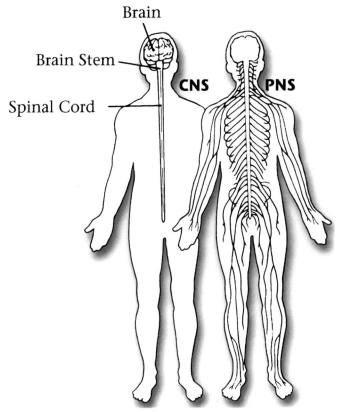

Brain

Brain Stem

Spinal Cord

CNS   PNS

Figure 2–1   The central nervous system (left) consists of the brain and spinal cord; the peripheral nervous system comprises the vast network of nerves that connect the brain and spinal cord to the rest of the body. (Courtesy of Harriet Greenfield. Reprinted by permission.)

with NF2 also develops some of the features that characterize NF1, notably skin tumors and café-au-lait spots. As Table **2–2** makes clear, however, the manifestations of NF1 and NF2 are sufficiently different that the two can be distinguished by careful physical examination and testing.

◆ The Variability Factor

Manifestations and their severity vary greatly in all three forms of neurofibromatosis. Although the *NF1* and *NF2* genes have been identified, the link between those genes and the physical manifestations of the

Table 2–2   Distinguishing Similar Features of NF1 and NF2

Features of NF1	How Such Features Appear in NF2
Six or more café-au-lait spots	One or two café-au-lait spots (always less than six)
Multiple Lisch nodules	Not seen
Multiple dermal neurofibromas	May have only a few dermal tumors. Biopsy will reveal these skin tumors to be schwannomas, not neurofibromas.
Spinal cord neurofibromas may occur	Spinal cord tumors may occur, and physical examination or MRI will not be able to distinguish them from neurofibromas. Biopsy, however, reveals that these are schwannomas.
Cognitive problems and learning disabilities are common	Not associated with NF2

disorder—what scientists call the *genotype-phenotype correlation*—is not well established in NF1 and predictive only in inherited cases of NF2. Although the mechanism causing schwannomatosis remains unknown, the disorder presents with varying degrees of severity. This "variability factor" is among the most worrisome aspects of living with neurofibromatosis.

In NF1, manifestations can vary by type and severity in the same family, as well as from one unrelated person to the next, or even in the same person over the course of a lifetime. It is also impossible so far to predict disorder severity in offspring. A parent with mild manifestations may have a child with severe manifestations. Likewise, a parent who has faced many complications from NF1 may have a child whose disorder is not severe. It is not clear what causes such variation in NF1 manifestations, but researchers suspect that factors such as hormones or other genes may be at work.

One exception to this general rule of heterogeneity in NF1 is a large deletion phenotype found in many, but not all, people who are missing the entire *NF1* gene. People with such deletions tend to develop a large number of dermal neurofibromas in childhood and suffer from mental retardation or developmental delays.[4–9]

In inherited NF2, there is a strong genotype-phenotype correlation, so that people in the same family tend to experience the same degree of severity. Even so, there may be some variation in such things as age of onset and the type of tumors that develop. In sporadic cases of NF2, it is more difficult to predict how severe manifestations will become. Some types of *mutations* have been associated with more medical complications, but genetic testing is not yet easily available or sensitive enough to predict phenotype.

Most cases of schwannomatosis arise spontaneously in people with no family history of neurofibromatosis. There is no way to predict the severity of symptoms.

As more is learned about the relationship between particular mutations and manifestations, it may be possible to provide a better genotype-phenotype correlation in neurofibromatosis. In the meantime, experience helps to predict when typical manifestations of neurofibromatosis are likely to occur. Not only does this assist in watchful waiting, but it also can enable people who are worried about specific manifestations to know when they can stop worrying.

◆ Living with Neurofibromatosis: The Personal Perspective

This chapter and many of those that follow provide the personal stories of people who have been diagnosed with neurofibromatosis, or have a loved one who has been. In their own words, they will provide their own perspective on these disorders, their diagnosis and treatment, and challenges and coping methods.

Nancy B. (Fig. **2–2**) is 50 years old, married, and works in computer science. She and her twin sister both have NF1.

"I have a fairly mild case. I wasn't diagnosed until I was about 18 years old. After my diagnosis, I didn't really think about NF again until my early thirties. Then I saw an article in the paper about a woman and her daughter who was severely affected. That article motivated me to learn more about NF and get more involved in the efforts to find a cure for it."

Porter C. (Fig. **2–3**) is 76 years old and retired. She worked as a medical secretary, laboratory technician, electrocardiogram technician, and medical records librarian. Two cats, Harry and Bob (Bob has a bobtail), live with her. She has NF1.

"When some parents of a child with NF see me, they say, 'My God, will my daughter or son look like that?' I tell them, 'Not necessarily. It's variable. The outcome is uncertain.' Life is real, like it or not. It's important to think positively. I feel the more tumors I have, the more of me there is to love."

Kellie C. (Fig. **2–4**) is 37 years old, a homemaker, and the mother of two children. She has NF1.

"I found out I had NF1 when I was a small child. I have a mild case. I have some neurofibromas, but not a lot. They're on my back and legs. My husband and I have been married since 1995. We wanted children. We're happy with the decision to have them."

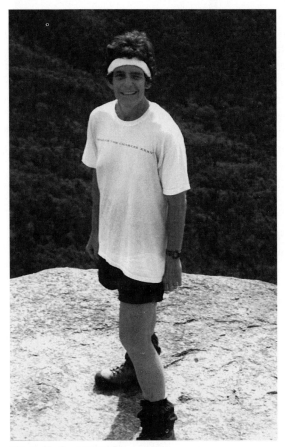

Figure 2–2   Nancy B.

Diane D. is an audiologist who is married and has two daughters. Julie (Fig. **2–5**), who just turned 9, has NF1. She is believed to be the first member of the family to have NF.

"Julie has had some challenges that are unusual. But that's the way it is with NF1. Anything goes. You don't know what might hit you. She has multiple café-au-lait spots and freckling. So far she has no neurofibromas. Julie seems so typical. She looks so normal, sometimes people doubt that she's got challenges. A lot of the problems are invisible."

Dolores G. raised three children. One of them, Susan (Fig. **2–6**), passed away in 2002 from complications of NF1. She was 34 years old. Dolores is a retired geriatric social worker.

"In her short life, Susan probably had about 40 major and minor surgeries. Her neurofibromas grew everyplace, on her feet, on her hands, and on her arms. She had a lot of them in the scalp, above her eye, and

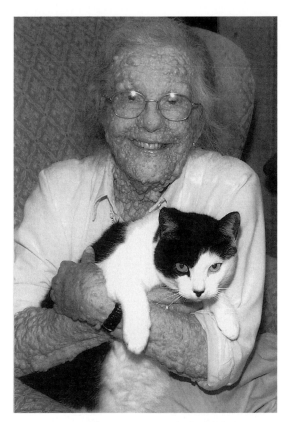

Figure 2–3 Porter C. (Courtesy of Scott Proposki. Reprinted by permission.)

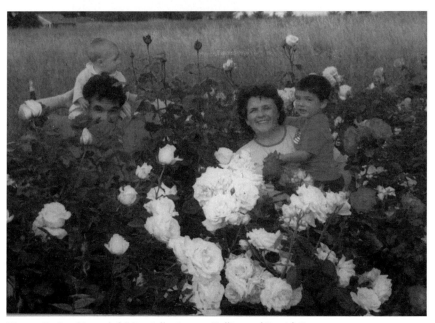

Figure 2–4 (From left) Danielle, James, Kellie, and David C.

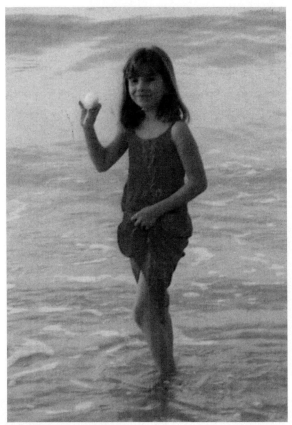

Figure 2–5   Julie D.

embedded in the eyebrow area, which caused headaches. She also had learning disabilities and developed plexiform neurofibromas."

Adam G. (Fig. **2–7**) is 18 years old, a senior in high school, and has been accepted on early admission into an Ivy League college. He wants to become a rabbi. Adam has NF2.

"Sometimes I think it would be nice if everyone knew what NF2 is, if NF2 were a household term. But then I think, if they taught it, they'd teach what it does at its most severe. Every disorder has mild as well as severe manifestations."

Marcy H. (Fig. **2–8**) passed away in 2003 at the age of 50. She was a former teacher, married, and a mother of two children. Marcy had schwannomatosis.

"Schwannomatosis is such an all-encompassing disorder. The tumors grow on the inside; nobody sees them. I feel like wearing a sign to let

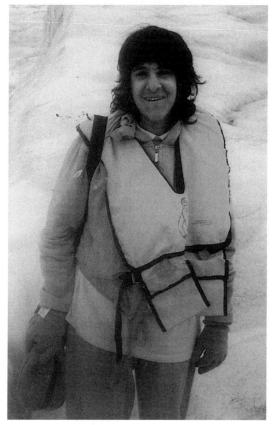

Figure 2–6   Susan G.

people know I have a disease. Because if people don't see it, they don't believe it exists."

Martha L. (Fig. **2–9**) is 34 years old, married, and works as an ultrasound technologist. She has NF2.

"It's been 15 years since I was diagnosed. In that time, I have lost most of my hearing. I also have many NF tumors in my brain, along my spine, and on other parts of my body. None of them are noticeable, except one on my finger. I have had to have some very major surgeries along with some minor ones because of these tumors."

Tamra M. (Fig. **2–10**) is 16 years old and in her junior year of high school. She plans to attend college and would like to become a writer. She has NF1.

"I'm very optimistic about the future, and I'll do whatever I want. I am not going to let NF get in my way. It's possible that other people's view of NF might, though. I think it's very important that people realize that it's

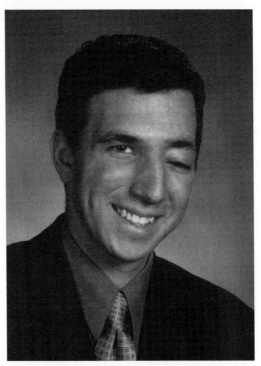

Figure 2–7   Adam G.

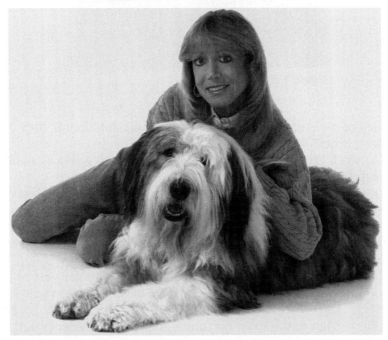

Figure 2–8   Marcy H. (Copyright 2003 Michael Lichterman/Clifford Norton Studio. Reprinted by permission.)

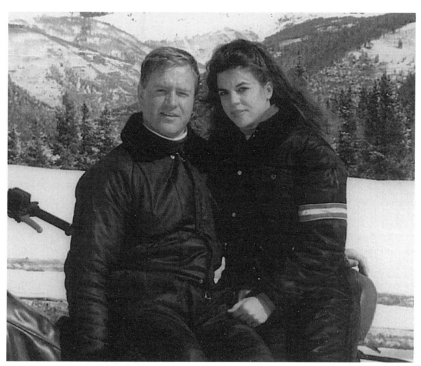

Figure 2–9   Martha and Gerry L.

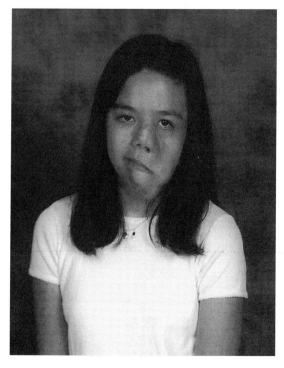

Figure 2–10   Tamra M.

not what is on the outside that counts, it's what is on the inside. I've been saying that since I was 7."

Angela W. (not pictured) is a 23-year-old homemaker who is married and has an 8-month-old son, Davin. She has NF1.

"I'm the first person in my family to have NF1. I have a mild case. I've had very few symptoms. I have a mild case of scoliosis, but that runs in the family anyway, so I'm not sure it's related to NF1. I've had minor learning disabilities. I have some café-au-lait spots, but I never had too many neurofibromas."

References

1. Gutmann DH, Aylsworth A, Carey JC, et al. The diagnostic evaluation and multidisciplinary management of neurofibromatosis 1 and neurofibromatosis 2. JAMA 1997;278:51–57

2. National Institutes of Health. NIH. Neurofibromatosis Consensus Development Conference. Neurofibromatosis Conference Statement. Arch Neurol 1988;45:575–578

3. National Institutes of Health Conference. Neurofibromatosis 1 (Recklinghausen disease) and neurofibromatosis 2 (bilateral acoustic neurofibromatosis): An update. Ann Intern Med 1990; 113:39–52

4. Kayes LM, Burke W, Riccardi VM, et al. Deletions spanning the neurofibromatosis 1 gene: identification and phenotype of five patients. Am J Hum Genet 1994;54:424–436

5. Leppig KA, Viskochil D, Neil S, et al. The detection of contiguous gene deletions at the neurofibromatosis 1 locus with fluorescence in situ hybridization. Cytogenet Cell Genet 1996;72:95–98

6. Leppig KA, Kaplan P, Viskochil D, Weaver M, Ortenberg J, Stephens K. Familial neurofibromatosis 1 microdeletions: co-segregation with distinct facial phenotype and early onset of cutaneous neurofibromata. Am J Med Genet 1997;73:197–204

7. Upadhyaya M, Ruggieri M, Maynard J, et al. Gross deletions of the neurofibromatosis type 1 (NF1) gene are predominantly of maternal origin and commonly associated with a learning disability, dysmorphic features and developmental delay. Hum Genet 1998;102:591–597

8. Wu BL, Austin MA, Schneider GH, Boles RG, Korf BR. Deletion of the entire NF1 gene detected by FISH: four deletion patients associated with severe manifestations. Am J Med Genet 1995;59:528–535

9. Wu BL, Schneider GH, Korf BR. Deletion of the entire NF1 gene causing distinct manifestations in a family. Am J Med Genet 1997;69:98–101

3

The Pathogenesis of Neurofibromatosis 1 and Neurofibromatosis 2

The neurofibromatoses are genetic disorders. NF1 and NF2 are each caused by a mutation in a known specific gene. The quest to understand how these disorders originate and progress (their *pathogenesis*) received a significant boost when researchers identified the causative genes. The leading theories about the pathogenesis of NF1 and NF2 are discussed in this chapter. Because the search for the biological cause of schwannomatosis was still underway when this book went to press, less is known about its pathogenesis (see Chapter 12).

◆ A Search for Answers

In 1990, two groups of scientists working separately located the *NF1* gene on chromosome 17 and characterized its protein product, *neurofibromin*.[1-3] In 1993, another two teams working separately identified the *NF2* gene on chromosome 22; one named its protein "*merlin*"[4] and the other "*schwannomin*."[5] Once the genes were identified, work could begin on better understanding how mutations lead to tumor formation and other manifestations.

The search for answers, however, has been daunting. There is probably no single answer to the question, What causes NF1 and NF2? Just as these disorders cause various types of manifestations, so too there appear to be multiple molecular mechanisms at work.

When trying to understand the pathogenesis of a disorder, scientists may combine two techniques that approach the question from different directions. The traditional phenotypical approaches analyze the physical manifestations of the disorders, such as what cells are involved and how they function, and then work backward to determine what gene might cause these abnormalities. The genotypical approach tries to understand how genes function normally and how mutations lead to the physical manifestations of disease.

Many advances in knowledge about neurofibromatosis have occurred as a result of these scientific methods, but much more remains to be learned. Both the *NF1* and *NF2* genes are large, complex, and prone to mutation. The *NF1* gene has one of the highest mutation rates of all genes.[6] Even so, this is an exciting time in the field of neurofibromatosis. As research yields additional insights into the pathogenesis of NF1, NF2, and schwannomatosis, diagnosis and treatments will improve.

◆ Two Genes with Similar Functions

When the *NF1* and *NF2* genes were first identified, both were classified as *tumor suppressors*. Although such genes are probably best known for their ability to prevent tumors from forming, their primary role in the body is to regulate cell growth and division. In the years since the *NF1* and *NF2* genes were discovered, scientists have learned more about not only how they regulate cell growth, but also the additional functions they perform in the body.

Cells divide and proliferate by following an orderly and highly regulated process known as the cell cycle. The process is initiated by *mitogenic* signals (from the word *mitosis,* or division), which function a bit like on-and-off switches. When it receives such a signal, the cell initiates the cycle and copies its chromosomes, chemical structures that contain genes. After repairing any genetic errors, the cell then divides into two identical cells. When this process breaks down, cells divide out of control, crowding out other cells and forming tumors.

Oncogenes are normal cellular genes that when mutated can initiate this type of abnormal growth. These genes, which help cause a variety of *cancers*, act in a *dominant* fashion. Just one mutation, or genetic "hit," is enough to initiate the growth of a cancerous tumor. People with neurofibromatosis already have one malfunctioning gene at birth. Yet it may take years for tumors to develop, and these only rarely progress to malignancy.

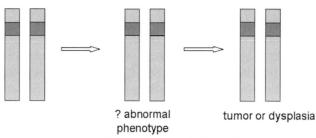

? abnormal   tumor or dysplasia
phenotype

Figure 3–1 According to the two-hit hypothesis, one functioning copy of a tumor suppressor gene is sufficient to regulate cell proliferation, even if the other copy is defective. Only when both copies of a tumor suppressor gene become inactivated do tumors form. (From Korf BR. Human Genetics: A Problem-Based Approach. Oxford: Blackwell Science; 2000:280, with permission.)

Scientists decided that the neurofibromatosis genes, therefore, seemed to conform to Alfred Knudson's "two-hit theory" about tumor suppressors (Fig. **3–1**). Knudson developed this hypothesis when describing the disease process that leads to retinoblastoma, a rare childhood cancer affecting the retina of the eye.[7,8] Retinoblastoma does not occur in neurofibromatosis; the two disorders are caused by different genes. Even so, the gene responsible for retinoblastoma (the *Rb* gene) formed the paradigm of the tumor suppressor model, which applies to both the *NF1* and *NF2* genes.

Although both the *NF1* and *NF2* genes function as tumor suppressors, they may inhibit cellular proliferation through different mechanisms. The *NF1* gene normally suppresses cell growth directly by regulating the response to mitogenic signals. The *NF2* gene works less directly, by regulating the function of signals sent between cells, and from cells to the surrounding matrix, which also inhibits or encourages cell proliferation. Both genes may also be modified or enhanced by *hormones* and the interaction with other genes, although this is an area deserving a great deal of rigorous study.

◆ Basic Genetics

NF1 and NF2 are both *autosomal dominant* disorders. Understanding what this means, and how these disorders develop, requires a basic knowledge of medical genetics. A brief introduction for the layperson is provided below. For information about why there is a 50/50 chance of passing NF1 and NF2 on to offspring, see Chapter 4.

What Genes Do

Each cell in the body contains 23 pairs of chromosomes. One member of a pair of chromosomes is inherited from the mother and the other from the father. Chromosomes 1 through 22 are known as autosomal chromosomes, and are the same in males and females. NF1 and NF2 are autosomal disorders because their genes are located on one of the autosomes. Chromosomes in the 23rd pair are known as the sex chromosomes (XX for females; XY for males).

Chromosomes are located in the cell's nucleus, which functions much like a command center that sends instructions to the rest of the cell. When genes are activated or expressed, they produce proteins that determine everything from physical characteristics, such as hair color, to less obvious traits, such as susceptibility to disease. Genes do this by providing molecular blueprints for proteins that perform various tasks. The blueprint is in the form of a unique sequence of DNA, the basic chemical building blocks of heredity (Fig. **3–2**).

Some genes are dominant and some are *recessive*—a concept first established by Gregor Mendel, the 19th century monk whose experiments

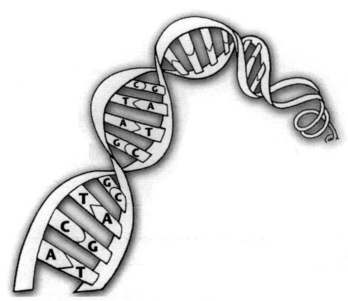

Figure 3–2   DNA is spelled out in code consisting of various combinations of four chemical bases, each represented by a letter: A (for adenine), T (thymine), G (guanine), and C (cytosine). A strand of DNA resembles a double helix. When DNA is copied, the two strands pull apart. (Courtesy of Harriet Greenfield, with permission.)

with plants led to his landmark discovery of patterns of heredity. (Mendel wondered why a tall plant cross-bred with a small plant did not produce offspring of medium height. That led to the insight that certain inherited traits were dominant. The way those traits are passed on through genes would not be discovered until the next century.) Although each person has two copies of every gene, it takes two recessive genes to produce a trait, but just one dominant gene. Both NF1 and NF2 are caused by a change in a dominant gene.

How Genes Mutate

Whenever a cell divides, it first makes a complete copy of its DNA to pass on to the daughter cell (Fig. **3–3**). Mutations can occur at any time during cell division, due to a simple copying error. Or an outside mutagen (something that can cause a mutation) such as a toxin might injure a cell's DNA. However it happens, the mutation then gets passed on the next time the cell divides.

When a DNA sequence changes because of a mutation, the genetic code gets scrambled. As a result, part of the instructions for the protein may be missing, or they may be arranged out of order. This causes some abnormality in the gene product. A truncated protein, for instance, does not contain all the necessary "ingredients" and functions poorly. At other times the protein cannot be made at all, or contains the wrong amino acid.

Researchers working on the Human Genome Project estimate that people have a total of 30,000 to 40,000 genes.[9] Because people inherit two copies of each gene, this means the nucleus of each cell contains about as many genes as there are words in this book. Both NF1 and NF2 develop

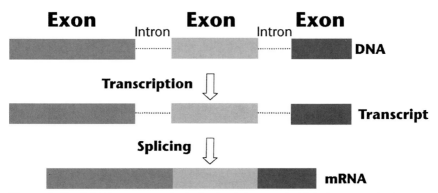

Figure 3–3   A DNA sequence includes both introns (which do not code for any-thing) and exons. The entire sequence is transcribed, but the introns are spliced out of the transcript to produce mature messenger RNA (mRNA). The cell uses mRNA to synthesize a protein. (From Korf BR. Human Genetics: A Problem-Based Approach. Oxford: Blackwell Science; 2000:27, with permission.)

from a mutation in just one gene (or, to use an analogy, an error in just one word in this book), which may then be exacerbated by mutations in additional "modifying" genes. The original error might be as small as the substitution of one chemical base for another in the genetic code (similar to a mistyped letter in one of the words you are reading), or as large as the deletion of the entire gene (similar to a single missing word).

From Genetic Error to Disorder

There are thousands of proteins in the body, which interact with one another to regulate basic cellular processes. When a genetic mutation causes one protein to malfunction, it can set off a domino-like chain reaction that affects other genes and proteins as well. Eventually this may cause manifestations of a disorder, such as tumor formation in neurofibromatosis. To determine the multiple biochemical steps between a single genetic error and the multiple manifestations of neurofibromatosis, scientists study *signaling pathways*—the sequence of individual genes and proteins (the dominos, if you will) that are activated or deactivated by the *NF1* and *NF2* genes.

To do this, scientists sometimes study actual tumor tissue taken from people with NF1 or NF2, which is then examined for telltale signs of genetic mutation. Another method is to conduct studies of living cells grown in the laboratory from donated samples (the in vitro approach). Or researchers may devise experiments in vivo, in living models of the disease, such as mice or fruit flies.

Generally scientists employ two techniques to better understand a gene's function. One method is to overexpress it so that it causes more dramatic, and thus more easily observed, effects than if it were expressed normally. Another approach is to create knockout models, animals or lower organisms that are genetically engineered to lack function of one or both copies of a gene. This enables researchers to determine what happens when one or both copies of the gene are absent. Both methods provide clues about the gene's normal function and what happens when it is mutated.

◆ The Pathogenesis of Neurofibromatosis 1

NF1 Gene Structure and Mutations

The *NF1* gene (Fig. **3–4**) consists of ~335,000 chemical bases,[10] making it one of the largest genes in the human body. Three of the gene's coding regions, known as *exons*, are alternatively spliced,[11-13] meaning that sometimes they are spliced in or out of the final translated sequence. This

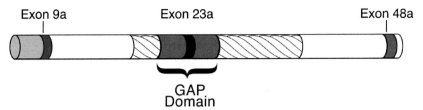

Figure 3–4 Diagram of the *NF1* gene, showing three alternatively spliced exons (9a, 23a, and 48a) and the GAP-related domain. GAP: guanosine triphosphatase activating protein. (From Gutmann DH. The neurofibromatoses: when less is more. Hum Mol Genet 2001;10:749, with permission.)

creates a slightly different protein or isoform. This is a fairly typical feature of genes and probably enables them to take on different functions in various areas of the body. The *NF1* gene also contains three "nested" but separate genes—known as *EVI2A*, *EVI2B*, and *OMGP*—that are embedded into one of its noncoding introns.[14(p120)] The function of these embedded genes is not known. Initially scientists speculated that they might have some effect on the manifestations of NF1 and might even help explain why manifestations can vary so greatly in people with the disorder. However, research in this area has been inconclusive so far.

Many different types of mutations, probably more than 500 at this point, have been identified in the *NF1* gene. The exact mutation usually differs from one person to the next, and only in a small number of cases have identical mutations been identified.

Categories of mutations identified to date are listed in Table **3–1**. Most of the mutations result in gross truncation (a shorter-than-normal version) of neurofibromin.[15] Whatever the type of *NF1* mutation, neurofibromin is either defective or available in such small quantities that it can't do its job correctly.

NF1 Gene Expression

Little is known at this point about what factors activate *NF1* gene expression,[16(p601)] but its protein product neurofibromin is expressed in several different cells throughout the body. The strongest expression is in cells of the nervous system,[16(p593)] including neurons and *glial cells* such as Schwann cells, oligodendrocytes, and astrocytes[17] (see Chapter 2). Neurofibromin is also expressed in cells derived from the *neural crest*, a structure that is created early in embryonic development and eventually gives rise to pigment cells in the skin, bone, and some components of the peripheral nervous system. Melanocytes, for instance, produce skin pigmentation. Many nervous system and neural crest cells, of course, are also those that develop abnormalities in people with NF1.

Table 3–1   Types of Gene Mutations in NF1

Mutation	Notes
Small deletion	Removal of a small number of DNA bases, usually leading to failure of protein production
Premature "stop" mutation	Changing the genetic instructions to insert an amino acid to a sequence that causes production of the protein to stop
Deletion of multiple exons	Can result in either shortening of the protein or complete failure of production
Amino acid substitution	May alter the structure or function of the protein
Small insertion	Has similar impact as small deletion
Mutation of an intron (noncoding section of a gene)	Interferes with the splicing process, resulting in an abnormal protein, or no protein produced at all
Deletion of entire gene	Complete gene deletion results in no protein product from that gene copy
Chromosome abnormality	A rearrangement of the structure of a chromosome can disrupt a gene, such as *NF1*
Alteration of the 3' untranslated region	Unclear if changes that follow the coding sequence of the *NF1* gene are really mutations or incidental changes
Large insertion	Has similar impact as large deletions

Impact on the Cell Cycle

The two prevailing theories about the pathogenesis of NF1 have something in common: that loss of the gene's protein product somehow disrupts the normal sequence of signals responsible for controlling cell division. To appreciate how even subtle errors in molecular signaling pathways can wreak such havoc, it is important to understand the basics of the cell cycle, which initiates and controls cell division.

The cell cycle is an orderly four-step process that ends when the cell divides into two daughter cells. The cycle is regulated by a network of signaling molecules that respond to information both within and outside the cell. To use a familiar analogy, these signaling molecules are the biological versions of air traffic controllers. Some molecules monitor the status of a cell (similar to keeping an eye on a single plane); others monitor the environment (the sky or the runway). A series of signals are sent for the cell to divide (or the plane to land) only when the cell is ready and the conditions right (landing gear down, and runway clear). Otherwise, the cell will receive another set of signals that act as brakes that stop the cycle at various checkpoints. This may occur if something goes wrong during the process, or if it is simply not yet time to divide. These controls on the cycle ensure that cells wait their turn to divide and do not crowd out neighbors. Neurofibromin appears to act as a molecular brake, which is why its loss enables the cell to proliferate out of control.

NF1 Gene Signaling Pathways

Researchers are still trying to determine all of neurofibromin's functions. Part of the challenge is the sheer size of the protein. Another is the complexity and interdependence of cells in the nervous system, which makes it difficult at times to determine which manifestations of NF1 are caused by loss of neurofibromin and which are caused by other factors. A third challenge is developing models in animals and lower organisms that mimic manifestations of NF1. Mice genetically engineered to have one functioning and one defective *NF1* gene, to mimic the genetics of the disorder, do not develop tumors typical of NF1. Experiments in chimeric mice, bred to contain a defective *NF1* gene as well as other features of the disorder, are helping researchers to create more accurate animal models of the disorder. Also useful are "conditional knockout" mice, in which both copies of the *NF1* gene can be switched off by the investigator.

In spite of these challenges, researchers have gained much insight into neurofibromin's functions by tracing the series of biochemical events that are triggered when the *NF1* gene is expressed. This has helped researchers to learn what happens when the gene is mutated.

The Ras-GAP Pathway

The prevailing theory about how neurofibromin functions in the body is that it behaves like a guanosine triphosphatase (GTPase)-activating protein (GAP). Members of the GAP family regulate other proteins, including one known as *Ras,* which is the specific target for neurofibromin GAP activity. There are more than 50 members in the Ras family,[14(p126)] and these proteins are best known for their role in initiating cell proliferation.[18(p14)] Several studies suggest that Ras also has a role in cell differentiation—the process by which cells develop specialized functions.[19,20] This means that neurofibromin interaction with Ras may have an impact not only on tumor growth but also on basic development.[16(p594)]

Researchers first suspected that neurofibromin might regulate Ras when they noticed that a small segment of the *NF1* gene resembles the sequence of genes in the GAP family.[21(p748)] Several functional studies have shown that neurofibromin does indeed regulate Ras.[16(p593)] Neurofibromin serves to act as a brake on cell proliferation, whereas Ras functions more as a gas pedal. The two are constantly in play to keep cell growth and

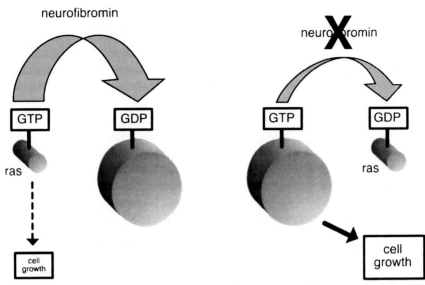

Figure 3–5   When Ras binds to a molecule known as guanosine triphosphate (GTP), it becomes active and promotes cell growth. When neurofibromin functions normally, the GTP is converted to guanosine diphosphate (GDP), which inactivates Ras so that cell growth is held in check. When neurofibromin expression is compromised (as it is in people who have a mutation in the *NF1* gene), Ras remains active and promotes cell proliferation and tumor growth. (From Gutmann DH. The neurofibromatoses: when less is more. Hum Mol Genet 2001;10:749, with permission.)

proliferation balanced and under control. But when the *NF1* gene is mutated, there is not enough neurofibromin to counter the actions of Ras. The result is out-of-control cell growth and tumor formation (Fig. **3–5**).

Ras activation, and neurofibromin regulation, may be involved in more than tumor formation. Recent research also indicates that Ras overexpression in the brain may contribute to the *learning disabilities* that are common in people with NF1 (see Chapter 8).

Although questions remain about exactly how neurofibromin regulates Ras, the fact that overactive Ras expression is linked to many manifestations of NF1 provides fertile ground for research. As scientists learn more about the pathophysiology of NF1, and what role Ras and other molecules play, new targets for therapy may be identified.

The cAMP-PKA Pathway

The GAP-related domain of the *NF1* gene comprises only 10% of its entire coding region.[21(p749)] This suggests that the gene may have other functions besides regulating the Ras pathway.[16(p601)] One of the other signaling pathways that neurofibromin may regulate is known as the cAMP-PKA pathway (short for cyclic adenosine 3',5'-monophosphate–protein kinase A). Some of the strongest evidence for this theory comes from experiments done in fruit flies, which suggest that neurofibromin regulation of the cAMP-PKA pathway influences the action of neurons in the brain and may provide another mechanism through which neurofibromin defects contribute to NF1 learning disabilities[18(p16)] (see Chapter 8).

Experiments in mice have indicated that a reduction in neurofibromin levels affects how responsive Schwann cells are to cAMP. This is significant because an overproliferation of Schwann cells contributes to neurofibroma formation in NF1. Although scientists are still trying to connect all the dots, it is thought that neurofibromin loss, PKA signaling, and levels of cAMP are somehow related.[21(p749)] Although the research continues, it may be that neurofibromin regulates cell proliferation and other cell activities not only by working through the Ras pathway, but also by working through the cAMP-PKA pathway, and possibly other cell signaling pathways.

◆ How *NF1* Gene Mutations May Cause Manifestations

As mentioned earlier in this chapter, a leading theory is that the *NF1* gene functions as a tumor suppressor. That gives rise to the questions of how it regulates cell growth, and why a mutation leads to tumor growth in NF1. Several mechanisms of action have been proposed, depending on the type of tumor.

Just why manifestations develop depends in part on whether one or both copies of the *NF1* gene are mutated. If both copies of the *NF1* gene are mutated (the "second hit" in Knudson's tumor suppressor theory), the resulting loss of neurofibromin leads to abnormal cell growth following the classic tumor suppressor model. Second hits are evident in tissue taken from malignant tumors in NF1 patients, such as *pheochromocytomas* and *malignant peripheral nerve sheath tumors*,[22–24] as well as in benign neurofibromas. Other evidence suggests that a reduction in neurofibromin to less-than-normal levels (a situation known as *haploinsufficiency*) may contribute to many nontumor manifestations of NF1, such as café-au-lait spots, bone deformities, and cognitive impairments.[16(p601)]

To further complicate the picture, factors such as hormones and other genes may themselves modify or enhance neurofibromin's own effects in cells. This would help to explain why manifestations of NF1 vary so much, even among siblings who inherit the same genetic mutation.[16(p593)] This theory is attractive because tumors tend to form only after multiple "hits" to various genes. Many cancers, for instance, involve the loss of a DNA repair mechanism, the transformation of a normal gene into an oncogene, and the malfunctioning of a tumor suppressor gene. Still another reason for variability is chance: severity of manifestations may depend on whether a second hit occurs in a given nerve at a specific time during development.

◆ Pathogenesis of Tumors

Neurofibromas

One of the most common manifestations in NF1, the growth of neurofibromas, is also one of the most complicated. Both *dermal neurofibromas* and *plexiform neurofibromas* consist of the many cells normally found in peripheral nerve tissue. An individual nerve is made up of multiple cells: peripheral neurons, Schwann cells, and cells in the surrounding area such as fibroblasts, endothelial cells, and mast cells. These cells are all bundled into fascicles and then surrounded by layers of perineural cells. Yet this very commingling and interdependence has made it difficult to untangle the process of tumor formation in neurofibromas.

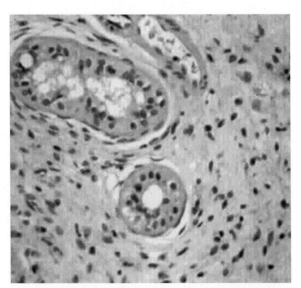

Figure 3–6 Photomicrograph of neurofibroma showing varied cell types. (Courtesy of Dr. Harry Kozakewich, Children's Hospital Boston, with permission.)

When scientists analyze tissue from different NF1 tumor types, they find evidence of loss of heterozygosity (the "second hit") in malignant peripheral nerve sheath tumors, which develop from plexiform neurofibromas; second hits are also evident in benign neurofibromas.[25-30] Development of genetically engineered chimeric mice have provided an animal model showing that loss of heterozygosity is required for neurofibroma formation.[31] Subsequent research revealed that a "second hit" in a Schwann cell is the initiating event, but that neurofibromas form only if there is NF1 haploinsufficiency in surrounding cells.[32] These other cells may be responsive to the aberrant cell's signaling or may be sensitive to the specific loss of neurofibromin.[16(p596)]

In any event, neurofibroma formation is a coordinated process that involves not only the initiating Schwann cell but also neighboring cells. As the Schwann cell begins to divide abnormally, it influences other Schwann cells (which seem particularly sensitive to neurofibromin levels) as well as other supportive cells: perineural cells, mast cells, fibroblasts, and neurons (Figs. **3–6** and **3–7**). When the perineural cells become involved, they not only proliferate in excess but also disrupt the diffusion barrier, a sort of protective structure that keeps circulating hormones and growth factors at bay. Once the barrier is disrupted, however, these molecules can themselves encourage more cell growth, only further fueling the out-of-control proliferation.

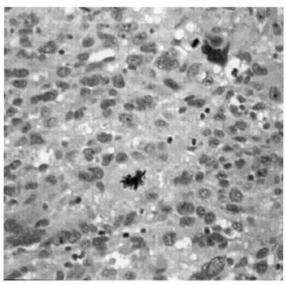

Figure 3–7 Photomicrograph of malignant peripheral nerve sheath tumor showing varied cell types. (Courtesy of Dr. Harry Kozakewich, Children's Hospital Boston, with permission.)

Optic Gliomas

Gliomas are tumors that develop from glial cells in the brain. Typically these are benign and develop on the optic nerve leading from the eye to the brain. It is not yet clear what factors contribute to the development of gliomas, but neurofibromin appears to play a role, albeit one that is slightly different from its contribution to neurofibroma development.

One theory is that neurofibromin loss somehow initiates tumor development—a theory that is supported by laboratory experiments that show that when one *NF1* gene is mutated, thereby reducing neurofibromin expression, astrocyte proliferation increases.[33–35] Another theory is that gliomas develop because neurofibromin loss in these cells disrupts the normal response to injury. Although normally expressed at low levels in astrocytes, neurofibromin is sometimes overexpressed in response to an injury that interrupts blood flow to the brain (known medically as ischemia).[36] If the *NF1* gene is defective, however, neurofibromin may not be able to function, and enzymes and cells released during an inflammatory response may themselves spark astrocytoma proliferation.[16(p600)]

Malignant Peripheral Nerve Sheath Tumors

Five to ten percent of people with NF1 develop malignant peripheral nerve sheath tumors (MPNSTs), which are believed to originate for the most part in plexiform neurofibromas.[37] Analysis of tissue from these tumors indicates that in addition to sustaining mutations in both copies of the *NF1* gene, additional mutations and second hits have been sustained by other genes, primarily the *p53* tumor suppressor gene[38,39] and two other tumor suppressors, *p16INK4a* and *p14ARF*.[40–42] Taken together with studies in mice, the evidence suggests that *p53* and the *NF1* genes must both be completely inactivated and then spark a cascade of other biological events that initiate MPNST development.[16(p599)] It may well be that other genes interact with the *NF1* gene to create malignancies in people with NF1.

◆ Additional Physical Manifestations

The earliest manifestations of NF1 include café-au-lait spots, *skinfold freckling*, and Lisch nodules. All of these manifestations involve abnormalities of cells derived from the neural crest early in embryonic development. Abnormalities in melanocytes, for instance, contribute to the darker pigmentation in both café-au-lait spots and Lisch nodules. The chromaffin cells, located in the adrenal medulla (part of the endocrine system), sometimes give rise to pheochromocytomas.

Laboratory experiments have shown that cells derived from the neural crest are sensitive to fluctuations in neurofibromin. They behave aberrantly, even under conditions of haploinsufficiency, when one *NF1* gene is mutated. Sometimes the effects are indirect. Studies in mice, for instance, suggest that reduced levels of neurofibromin have other downstream effects that can cause changes in coat color.[43]

◆ Theories of Pathogenesis in NF2

NF2 Gene Structure, Mutations, and Expression

The *NF2* gene (Fig. **3–8**) consists of 110,000 chemical bases.[14(p351)] The gene encodes for a protein that one team named "merlin" (for moesin-, ezrin- and radixin-like protein).[4] The other team called the protein "schwannomin" because, when it functions normally, it prevents the development of the hallmark NF2 tumor.[5] Two different versions of the NF2 protein can be produced, depending on circumstances and location in the body, because one exon is alternatively spliced.[14(p351)]

Many different types of mutations have been identified in the *NF2* gene, across most exons in the gene. These are summarized in Table **3–2**. There is no one "hot" spot where mutations occur more frequently than in other areas. Most inherited mutations have the effect of truncating the protein in one of several ways,[14(p353)] resulting in significant reduction in protein available to cells. The *NF2* gene is expressed throughout the body in many different types of cells, including neurons and glial cells such as Schwann cells, fibroblasts, and meningioma cells.[44–46]

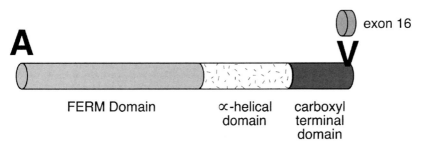

exon 16

A

FERM Domain   α-helical domain   carboxyl terminal domain

Figure 3–8 The *NF2* gene. FERM: Band 4.1, ezrin, radixin, moesin proteins. (From Gutmann DH. The neurofibromatoses: when less is more. Hum Mol Genet 2001;10:751, with permission.)

Table 3-2   Mutations in the *NF2* Gene

Type of Mutation	Frequency
Premature translation stop	38% of mutations
Reading frame shift, deletions, complex rearrangements	28%
Errors in splicing	24%
Insertions, deletions, amino acid substitutions (do not truncate protein)	10%

Adapted from MacCollin M, Gusella JF. Molecular biology. In: Friedman JM, Gutmann DH, MacCollin M, Riccardi VM, eds. Neurofibromatosis: Phenotype, Natural History, and Pathogenesis. 3rd ed. Baltimore: Johns Hopkins University Press; 1999:354, with permission.

NF2 Gene Signaling Pathways

Although the *NF2* gene is classified as a tumor suppressor, its protein product appears to regulate cell proliferation indirectly, by affecting cell-to-cell signals, and by the interaction between cells and surrounding tissue known as the extracellular matrix. The gene also appears to activate and interact with several signaling pathways.

Insights into merlin's function started when researchers realized that the *NF2* gene sequence resembles members of a family of proteins that affect the interactions of cells and the cytoskeleton, a complex set of structures within the cell. This family includes erythrocyte protein 4.1, moesin, ezrin, radixin, and talin, none of which is associated with regulation of cell proliferation or tumor formation. Instead, these proteins regulate interactions with the cytoskeleton to determine cell shape, movement, division, and cell-to-cell communication. This finding was unexpected, and it suggested that the *NF2* gene might represent a new type of tumor suppressor.[4]

Although merlin interacts with several other proteins, its signaling pathways have not yet been well defined. One theory is that merlin may interact with another protein, known as Expanded (a member of the 4.1 protein family), to control cell proliferation.[47] Another theory is that the *NF2* gene may function as a "gatekeeper" gene that helps to regulate basic functions in a cell, such as division and proliferation, differentiation, and programmed cell suicide or apoptosis.[21(pp751,752)] Presumably, then, a mutation in the *NF2* gene, which causes a defect in or loss of its protein product, might result in a disruption of the normally harmonious interactions between cells, and between cells and the surrounding matrix. This could, in turn, indirectly disrupt cellular proliferation.[5(p521)] Normally cells continue to divide, for instance, until they encounter other cells—a phenomenon known as contact inhibition. If this inhibition were lost because the *NF2* gene caused disruptions in the cell-matrix communication network, then these cells would begin to multiply out of control.

◆ How *NF2* Gene Mutations May Cause Tumors

In addition to the inherited *NF2* gene mutation, researchers have also found additional "second hits" to the gene in tumor tissue from people with the disorder. This confirms that the *NF2* gene functions as a tumor suppressor and that tumor formation is initiated when it is mutated. However, in some types of tumors, other genes or factors may participate in the process.

Schwannomas

Bilateral vestibular schwannomas affect almost everyone with NF2, although sometimes the tumors develop in only one ear. Analysis of schwannoma tumor tissue reveals that, as expected, both copies of the *NF2* gene are mutated in all samples taken from people with the familial form of NF2. Both copies of the gene are also mutated in schwannomas in most people with the sporadic form of the disorder.[21(p752)] Clearly, then, merlin functions as a tumor suppressor that prevents the development of schwannomas.

Meningiomas

These brain tumors occur less frequently than schwannomas in people with NF2, but they are the second most common type of tumor in the disorder. Double-hit *NF2* gene mutations are found in all meningiomas taken from people with the familial form of the disorder, and in 30 to 70% of sporadic meningiomas.[21(p752)] At least one study has reported, however, that some familial meningiomas do not show evidence of a second hit to the *NF2* gene, suggesting that some other tumor suppressor gene may prevent these tumors from forming.[48]

Other Tumors

Less is known about the status of *NF2* mutations in other types of NF2-related tumors, such as *ependymomas, astrocytomas,* and *gliomas.* The research in this area continues.

References

1. Cawthon RM, Weiss R, Xu G, et al. A major segment of the neurofibromatosis type 1 gene: cDNA sequence, genomic structure, and point mutations. Cell 1990;62:193–201
2. Viskochil D, Buchberg AM, Xu G, et al. Deletions and a translocation interrupt a cloned gene at the neurofibromatosis type 1 locus. Cell 1990;62:187–192
3. Wallace MR, Marchuk DA, Andersen LB, et al. Type 1 neurofibromatosis gene: identification of a large transcript disrupted in three NF1 patients. Science 1990;249:181–186
4. Trofatter JA, MacCollin M, Rutter JL, et al. A novel moesin-, ezrin-, radixin-like gene is a candidate for the neurofibromatosis 2 tumor suppressor. Cell 1993;72:791–800
5. Rouleau GA, Merel P, Lutchman M, et al. Alteration in a new gene encoding a putative membrane-organizing protein causes neurofibromatosis type 2. Nature 1993;363:515–521
6. Viskochil DH. Gene structure and expression. In: Upadhyaya M, Cooper DN, eds. Neurofibromatosis Type 1: From Genotype to Phenotype. Oxford: BIOS Scientific Publishers; 1998:39–53. Cited by: Ruggieri M, Huson SM. The clinical and diagnostic implications of mosaicism in the neurofibromatoses. Neurology 2001;56:1433
7. Knudson AG Jr. Mutation and cancer: statistical study of retinoblastoma. Proc Natl Acad Sci USA 1971;68:820–823
8. Knudson AG Jr, Hethcote HW, Brown BW. Mutation and childhood cancer: a probabilistic model for the incidence of retinoblastoma. Proc Natl Acad Sci USA 1975;72:5116–5120
9. About the Human Genome Project. National Human Genome Research Institute Web site. Available at: http://www.genome.gov/10001772
10. Li Y, O'Connell P, Breidenbach HH, et al. Genomic organization of the neurofibromatosis 1 gene (NF1). Genomics 1995;25:9–18
11. Danglot G, Regnier V, Fauvet D, Vassal G, Kujas M, Bernheim A. Neurofibromatosis 1 (NF1) mRNAs expressed in the central nervous system are differentially spliced in the 5' part of the gene. Hum Mol Genet 1995;4:915–920
12. Andersen LB, Ballester R, Marchuk DA, et al. A conserved alternative splice in the von Recklinghausen neurofibromatosis (NF1) gene produces two neurofibromin isoforms, both of which have GTPase-activating protein activity. Mol Cell Biol 1993;13:487–495
13. Gutmann DH, Andersen LB, Cole JL, Swaroop M, Collins FS. An alternatively spliced mRNA in the carboxy terminus of the neurofibromatosis type 1 (NF1) gene is expressed in muscle. Hum Mol Genet 1993;2:989–992
14. Friedman JM, Gutmann DH, MacCollin M, Riccardi VM, eds. Neurofibromatosis: Phenotype, Natural History, and Pathogenesis. 3rd ed. Johns Hopkins University Press; 1999
15. Upadhyaya M, Cooper D. The mutational spectrum in neurofibromatosis 1 and its underlying mechanisms. In: Upadhyaya M, Cooper DN, eds. Neurofibromatosis Type 1: From Genotype to Phenotype. Oxford: BIOS Scientific Publishers; 1998. Cited by: Friedman JM, Gutmann DH, MacCollin M, Riccardi VM, eds. Neurofibromatosis: Phenotype, Natural History, and Pathogenesis. 3rd ed. Baltimore: Johns Hopkins University Press; 1999:127
16. Cichowski K, Jacks T. NF1 tumor suppressor gene function: narrowing the GAP. Cell 2001;104:593–604
17. Daston MM, Scrable H, Nordlund M, Sturbaum AK, Nissen LM, Ratner N. The protein product of the neurofibromatosis type 1 gene is expressed at highest abundance in neurons, Schwann cells, and oligodendrocytes. Neuron 1992;8:415–428
18. Weiss B, Bollag G, Shannon K. Hyperactive ras as a therapeutic target in neurofibromatosis type 1. Am J Med Genet 1999;89:14–22
19. Marshall CJ. Specificity of receptor tyrosine kinase signaling: transient versus sustained extra-cellular signal-regulated kinase activation. Cell 1995;80:179–185
20. Schlessinger J. Cell signaling by receptor tyrosine kinases. Cell 2000;103:211–225
21. Gutmann DH. The neurofibromatoses: when less is more. Hum Mol Genet 2001;10:747–755
22. Xu W, Mulligan LM, Ponder MA, et al. Loss of NF1 alleles in phaeochromocytomas from patients with type 1

neurofibromatosis. Genes Chromosomes Cancer 1992;4:337–342

23. Legius E, Marchuk DA, Collins FS, Glover TW. Somatic deletion of the neurofibromatosis type 1 gene in a neurofibrosarcoma supports a tumour suppressor gene hypothesis. Nat Genet 1993;3:122–126

24. Shannon KM, O'Connell P, Martin GA, et al. Loss of the normal NF1 allele from the bone marrow of children with type 1 neurofibromatosis and malignant myeloid disorders. N Engl J Med 1994;330:597–601

25. Colman SD, Williams CA, Wallace MR. Benign neurofibromas in type 1 neurofibromatosis (NF1) show somatic deletions of the *NF1* gene. Nat Genet 1995;11:90–92

26. Sawada S, Florell S, Purandare SM, Ota M, Stephens K, Viskochil D. Identification of *NF1* mutations in both alleles of a dermal neurofibroma. Nat Genet 1996;14:110–112

27. Serra E, Puig S, Otero D, et al. Confirmation of a double-hit model for the NF1 gene in benign neurofibromas. Am J Hum Genet 1997;61:512–519

28. Jessen KR, Mirsky R. Origin and early development of Schwann cells. Microsc Res Tech 1998;41:393–402

29. Kluwe L, Friedrich RE, Mautner VF. Alleic loss of the *NF1* gene in NF1-associated plexiform neurofibromas. Cancer Genet Cytogenet 1999; 113:65–69

30. Rasmussen SA, Overman J, Thomson SA, et al. Chromosome 17 loss-of-heterozygosity studies in benign and malignant tumors in neurofibromatosis type 1. Genes Chromosomes Cancer 2000;28:425–431

31. Cichowski K, Shane Shih T, Schmitt E, et al. Mouse models of tumor development in neurofibromatosis type 1. Science 1999;286:2172–2176

32. Zhu Y, Ghosh P, Charnay P, Burns DK, Parada LF. Neurofibromas in NF1: Schwann cell origin and role of tumor environment. Science 2002; 296:920–922

33. Lau N, Feldkamp MM, Roncari L, et al. Loss of neurofibromin is associated with activation of ras/MAPk and P13k/AKT signaling in a neurofibromatosis 1 astrocytoma. J Neuropathol Exp Neurol 2000;59:759–767

34. Nordlund ML, Rizvi TA, Brannan CI, Ratner N. Neurofibromin expression

and astrogliosis in neurofibromatosis (type 1) brains. J Neuropathol Exp Neurol 1995;54:588–600

35. Gutmann DH, Loehr A, Zhang Y, Kim J, Henkemeyer M, Cashen A. Haploinsufficiency for the neurofibromatosis 1 (NF1) tumor suppressor results in increased astrocyte proliferation. Oncogene 1999;18:4450–4459

36. Giordano MJ, Mahadeo DK, He YY, Geist RT, Hsu C, Gutmann DH. Increased expression of the neurofibromatosis 1 (NF1) gene product, neurofibromin, in astrocytes in response to cerebral ischemia. J Neurosci Res 1996;43:246–253

37. Woodruff JM. Pathology of the major peripheral nerve sheath neoplasms. In: Soft Tissue Tumors. International Academy of Pathology; 1996 Cited by: Cichowski K, Jacks T. NF1 tumor suppressor gene function: narrowing the GAP. Cell 2001;104:599

38. Menon AG, Anderson KM, Riccardi VM, et al. Chromosome 17p deletions and p53 gene mutations associated with the formation of malignant neurofibrosarcomas in von Recklinghausen neurofibromatosis. Proc Natl Acad Sci USA 1990;87:5435–5439

39. Greenblatt MS, Bennett WP, Hollstein M, Harris CC. Mutations in the p53 tumor suppressor gene: clues to cancer etiology and molecular pathogenesis. Cancer Res 1994;54:4855–4878

40. Berner JM, Sorlie T, Mertens F, et al. Chromosome band 9p21 is frequently altered in malignant peripheral nerve sheath tumors: studies of CDKN2A and other genes of the pRB pathway. Genes Chromosomes Cancer 1999;26:151–160

41. Kourea HP, Orlow I, Scheithauer BW, Cordon-Cardo C, Woodruff JM. Deletions of the INK4A gene occur in malignant peripheral nerve sheath tumors but not in neurofibromas. Am J Pathol 1999;155:1855–1860

42. Nielsen GP, Stemmer-Rachamimov AO, Ino Y, Moller MB, Rosenberg AE, Louis DN. Malignant transformation of neurofibromas in neurofibromatosis 1 is associated with CDKN2A/p16 inactivation. Am J Pathol 1999; 155:1879–1884

43. Ingram DA, Yang FC, Travers JB, et al. Genetic and biochemical evidence that haploinsufficiency of the *NF1* tumor suppressor gene modulates

melanocyte and mast cell fates in vivo. J Exp Med 2000;191:181–188

44. den Bakker MA, Riegman PH, Hekman RA, et al. The product of the NF2 tumour suppressor gene localizes near the plasma membrane and is highly expressed in muscle cells. Oncogene 1995;10:757–763

45. Scherer SS, Gutmann DH. Expression of the neurofibromatosis 2 tumor suppressor gene product, merlin, in Schwann cells. J Neurosci Res 1996;46:595–605

46. Stemmer-Rachamimov AO, Gonzalez-Agosti C, Xu L, et al. Expression of NF2 encoded merlin and related ERM family proteins in the human central nervous system. J Neuropathol Exp Neurol 1997;56:735–742

47. McCartney BM, Kulikauskas RM, LaJeunesse DR, Fehon RG. The neurofibromatosis-2 homologue, Merlin, and the tumor suppressor expanded function together in Drosophila to regulate cell proliferation and differentiation. Development 2000;127:1315–1324

48. Louis DN, Ramesh V, Gusella JF. Neuropathology and molecular genetics of neurofibromatosis 2 and related tumors. Brain Pathol 1995;5:163–172

4

Genetics and Genetic Counseling in Neurofibromatosis 1 and Neurofibromatosis 2

Molecular genetics explains how a mutation may cause a disorder. Clinical genetics takes a somewhat different perspective: how the mutation is inherited, how likely it is that the mutation will cause a disorder, and what medical and ethical decisions might face the patient and family. Some of the major components of clinical genetics, as it relates to neurofibromatosis 1 (NF1) and neurofibromatosis 2 (NF2), are explored in this chapter. (Schwannomatosis appears to have a hereditary pattern that is different from that of NF1 and NF2, and the biological mechanism that causes it is not yet known. For this reason, the issues of cause and genetic counseling are discussed in Chapter 12.)

◆ Common Questions About the Genetics of Neurofibromatosis 1 and Neurofibromatosis 2

What causes Neurofibromatosis 1 and Neurofibromatosis 2?

NF1 and NF2 both originate because of a change in a gene (i.e., the *NF1* or *NF2* gene). If a child with neurofibromatosis (NF) has a parent with NF, the condition has been inherited. If a child is diagnosed with the disorder but neither parent is affected, the condition probably developed because of a *spontaneous mutation* in an egg or sperm cell.

Can These Disorders Be Prevented?

At this time, there is no way to prevent NF1 or NF2. Genes mutate constantly in the body, and these genes have an unusually high rate of mutation, probably because both are relatively large and therefore there are more opportunities for error.

Many parents feel guilty when a child is diagnosed with NF, especially if there is no family history of the disorder. However, nothing a parent does (or doesn't do) can cause or prevent NF1 or NF2. These disorders are not caused by exposure to toxins, radiation exposure, or alcohol consumption.

What Is the Risk that a Parent Will Pass Neurofibromatosis on to the Child?

NF1 and NF2 are autosomal dominant conditions, which means that there is a 50/50 chance of passing the disorder on every time a person who has the disorder has a child.

Is Genetic Testing Available?

Genetic tests for NF1 and NF2 are now becoming available for routine clinical testing. These tests can be expensive, however, due to the complexity of finding the sometimes subtle mutations in the large *NF1* and *NF2* genes.

Is Genetic Therapy Available?

Currently gene therapy does not exist for NF1 and NF2. Scientists still have much work to do in understanding the basic disease process in both disorders before they will be able to develop interventions. In the meantime, many options exist for management.

◆ Principles of Autosomal Dominant Transmission

How Familial NF1 and NF2 Are Inherited

Once a person is born with the genetic mutation responsible for NF1 or NF2, there is a 50/50 chance of passing the condition on whenever that person has a child. To understand how offspring inherit these disorders, consider the principles of dominant inheritance.

Everyone has two copies of each gene. Most cells in the body hold both copies, contained in 46 chromosomes. The exceptions are egg and sperm cells, which contain only 23 chromosomes, and thus only one copy of each gene. When egg and sperm unite, 46 newly paired chromosomes result.

Thus, there are four possible genetic combinations every time egg and sperm unite (Fig. **4–1**). This explains why, for people who have NF, there is a 50% chance in every pregnancy for the child to have neurofibromatosis.

Obviously, the decision about whether or not to have a child can be difficult for someone with NF1 or NF2. The risk of passing the disorder on is akin to a coin toss, and yet the ramifications are much more serious. This is a decision that should be made carefully, and after consultations with the partner, other loved ones, a genetic counselor, and, for some people, a spiritual advisor. Both the *NF1* and *NF2* genes are highly penetrant, which means that if they are inherited they will cause manifestations. The real question is which manifestations and how severe those manifestations will be.

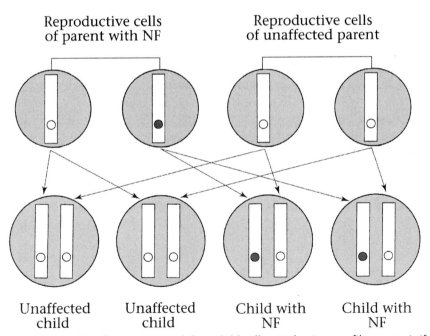

Reproductive cells of parent with NF

Reproductive cells of unaffected parent

Unaffected child

Unaffected child

Child with NF

Child with NF

Figure 4–1   Two illustrations on left: A child will not inherit neurofibromatosis if two unaffected reproductive cells unite. Two illustrations on right: A child will inherit the disorder if an affected cell is united with an unaffected cell. (Courtesy of Harriet Greenfield, with permission.)

Spontaneous Cases of Neurofibromatosis 1 and Neurofibromatosis 2

When NF1 or NF2 appears in a child born to parents who do not have the disorder, the typical reaction is: How could this happen? There are two possible answers. One is that a parent may in fact have NF1 or NF2, but the manifestations may be so mild that he or she does not realize it. The other explanation is that a mutation developed in either the sperm or egg cell that were joined at fertilization and eventually developed into the affected child.

Like other cells in the body, sperm and egg cells constantly divide as they develop and mature. Egg cells divide while a female fetus is still developing in the womb; consequently a woman is born with all the eggs she will ever have. Sperm cells continue dividing through a man's lifetime.

As discussed in Chapter 3, any time a cell divides there is a chance that a gene may mutate. Each time a cell divides, it first makes copies of thousands of genes, and there is always the chance that a copying error will occur sometime during the process. The genes that cause NF1 and NF2 are relatively large and therefore exceptionally prone to such copying errors. In fact, it is likely that most people have some egg or sperm cells that contain a mutated version of the *NF1* or *NF2* genes. When one egg or sperm cell containing a mutated *NF1* or *NF2* gene is involved in conception, the child who results will have the disorder.

When a sporadic case of NF1 or NF2 occurs, parents often wonder whether other children in the family will also have NF. In most cases, they will not, unless, by chance, there is another conception involving an egg or sperm with the requisite genetic mutation. It is unlikely (though not impossible) that parents who do not have NF will give birth to another child with NF1 or NF2. The child with NF, however, will have a 50/50 chance of giving birth to offspring with NF1 or NF2.

Mosaicism in Neurofibromatosis 1 and Neurofibromatosis 2

Although most sporadic cases of NF1 and NF2 occur when a chance mutation develops in either the sperm or egg cell that unite at conception to form a zygote, the resulting single fertilized cell, some occur because of a mutation that takes place later in prenatal development. Such *postzygotic mutations* develop into *mosaic* or *segmental* forms of neurofibromatosis. This person is born with a mixture of cells, some with two functioning copies of the *NF1* or *NF2* gene, and some with mutated copies (Fig. **4–2**).

If the postzygotic mutation occurs very early in embryonic development, before cells have begun to differentiate (take on specialized functions), most cells in the body will carry the mutation, and so the

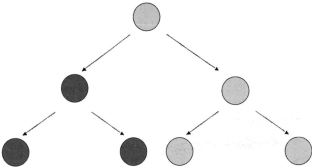

Figure 4–2   Mosaic forms of neurofibromatosis develop when a genetic mutation occurs during embryonic development. The child is born with a mixture of cells—some containing the NF mutation and some without. The condition is transmitted to offspring only when egg or sperm cells carry the mutation. (From Korf BR. Human Genetics: A Problem-Based Approach. Oxford: Blackwell Science; 2000:60, with permission.)

manifestations will be clinically indistinguishable from other cases of NF1 and NF2. If the postzygotic mutation occurs later in prenatal development, after cells have differentiated into different tissues and organs, manifestations may be milder or may result in only some parts of the body. An example of this is a case of NF2 where tumors develop in only one ear (known as *unilateral* vestibular schwannoma) and involve only one region of the body.[1] Another example, more controversial, is that of mosaic NF1, in which neurofibromas and pigmentary changes such as café-au-lait spots develop in only one area, such as one quadrant of the body.

The issue of mosaicism is probably of greater interest to genetic researchers than to patients and physicians. The condition can be confirmed only through genetic analysis of cells from different parts of the body. Clinically speaking, people with mosaic forms of NF1 and NF2 tend to have less severe manifestations, and they may be less likely to pass the disorder on to children. However, given the small likelihood that a case of spontaneous NF1 or NF2 is mosaic, and the difficulty in determining this, genetic counseling remains the same whether a person has the mosaic form or not.

◆ Genotype/Phenotype Correlations in NF1 and NF2

Genotype refers to a person's unique collection of genes, whereas *phenotype* refers to the physical characteristics that result when instructions from those genes are decoded. Both the *NF1* and *NF2* genes are prone to multiple types of mutations that affect manifestations of these disorders. There are no clear genotype-phenotype correlations in NF1; so far we cannot say which type of mutation can be linked to what type of clinical manifestation. The exceptions to this general rule are mutations that involve large or entire deletions of the gene. People with NF1 who have a large deletion mutation in the gene tend to develop neurofibromas earlier than expected, more significant developmental delays, and other physical anomalies.[2] In most cases, however, it is so far impossible to predict how mild or severe the disorder will be based on an analysis of the gene mutation or, in inherited cases, on the basis of other family members' manifestations.

On the other hand, there appear to be strong genotype/phenotype correlations in NF2. Members of the same family usually display the same manifestations and severity. It is possible, therefore, to predict with confidence how severe the manifestations of NF2 will be in people with the familial form of the disorder.

◆ Genetic Testing for Neurofibromatosis 1 and Neurofibromatosis 2

Genetic tests used in research may seek to characterize the type of mutation, determine whether it is inherited or acquired, and discover how the mutation affects the gene's protein product and an individual's physical characteristics, or phenotype. A variety of genetic tests exist for both NF1 and NF2, and in the research setting they have yielded many insights into the functioning of the *NF1* and *NF2* genes. (To learn more about how to participate in such research studies, see Chapter 15.)

Clinical genetic testing uses many of the same methods, but for a different reason: to determine whether someone has a gene mutation associated with a specific disorder. Clinical testing may be used to confirm a suspected diagnosis, or to establish the type of mutation as a prelude to offering prenatal diagnosis to a couple where one partner has the disorder. Because of the complexity of the *NF1* and *NF2* genes, genetic testing does not detect all possible mutations. The area of clinical genetic testing is changing rapidly, so consult your physician or a genetic counselor for up-to-date information.

Various types of genetic tests are available. Direct DNA testing examines the gene sequence segment by segment, and it provides the most specific information regarding the nature of a genetic mutation. This test predicts nothing about disorder severity. This method can be time consuming and expensive in large genes, such as *NF1* and *NF2*. A protein truncation test determines whether a gene's protein product (such as neurofibromin in NF1 or merlin in NF2) is altered in such a way that no protein or not enough protein is produced, which provides an indirect indication of whether a gene has mutated. The test is not specific enough to determine the particular mutation, however, unless it is followed by genetic sequencing. Fluorescence in situ hybridization (FISH) testing can determine whether the entire gene is deleted, but it is of value only to the small number of people who may have the "large deletion" NF1 phenotype. Linkage analysis takes DNA samples from affected and unaffected family members to track the manner by which the mutation is passed through the family. It is of value only to people who have the familial form of NF1. This type of testing requires not only that affected family members from three generations be available and willing to be tested, but also that the diagnosis be accurate in all those tested, and that genetic relationships be clear.

The decision about whether to obtain a genetic test can be difficult. Any type of genetic test has risks as well as benefits; thus the decision should be made only after weighing all the factors. Some guidance about the issues is provided in the section on genetic counseling.

Neurofibromatosis 1 Testing Issues

The chameleon nature of NF1 and the length of the *NF1* gene make genetic testing complicated. Such testing is now clinically available and can be used to confirm whether an *NF1* mutation is present in 95% of people tested. As mentioned earlier in this chapter, however, so far little is known about specific genotype-phenotype correlations in NF1, which means that even if a genetic mutation is detected in someone, it does not help a physician to predict what manifestations a person will experience. Moreover, genetic testing provides no information as yet that would serve to improve therapy in people with NF1. For these reasons, most cases of NF1 can be diagnosed and managed by a physician using the expert consensus clinical criteria (see Chapter 5).

Clinical Indications for Testing

There are two types of situations in which clinical genetic testing for the *NF1* gene mutation might be useful:

◆ **Confirming a Diagnosis**   In some unusual cases, a diagnosis of NF1 cannot be confirmed through any method other than a genetic test. The situation usually involves a child who develops multiple café-au-lait spots and is suspected of having NF1, yet is born with no family history of the disorder. In most situations, the best strategy is watchful waiting and conducting further clinical tests at the appropriate times (such as having the child examined by an ophthalmologist to detect the presence of Lisch nodules, which can be used to confirm a diagnosis). Because several years may pass before new signs of the disorder are discernible, parents sometimes become so anxious that it is difficult for them to wait. In this situation, a clinical genetic test could help to ease their anxiety by providing a definitive answer one way or the other. Another situation in which genetic testing might be helpful is when one of the parents has NF1 and a child displays minimal signs of having the disorder, such as four café-au-lait spots. In this case, testing may help determine whether the child has NF1. There are also times when a child or adult presents with unusual features of NF1, such as delayed onset of puberty or epilepsy, which may represent a variant form of the disorder. In this case, testing may help to clarify what is causing the manifestations.

◆ **Prenatal Testing**   It is possible to test a fetus for an *NF1* gene mutation if a parent has NF1 and is concerned about passing the disorder on to offspring. Samples of fetal DNA are obtained using either amniocentesis (a sample of the amniotic fluid surrounding the fetus, to detect any chromosomal abnormalities) or chorionic villus sampling (analysis of a tissue sample taken from the placenta to detect any genetic abnormalities). Direct analysis of fetal DNA is one possibility.[3] Linkage analysis provides another option for testing in people with the inherited form of NF1, as long as enough affected family members are available and willing to be tested.[4] As with adults, however, detecting a mutation does not predict how severely or mildly offspring will be affected; therefore, a genetic test is of no value in terms of prognosis. If parents request such testing to make a decision about whether or not to continue the pregnancy, then genetic counseling should be available so that they can make an informed decision.

Availability

Genetic tests for NF1 are now available on a clinical basis. Because of the large size of the *NF1* gene and the wide variety of possible mutations, it is difficult and costly to identify a particular mutation. A limited number of hospitals, universities, and diagnostic laboratories in the world provide such testing, and then only at the request of a physician (not a patient) and usually only for certain well-defined situations described above. In general, it is better to use clinical criteria for diagnosis and to monitor manifestations as they develop.

Neurofibromatosis 2 Testing Issues

Because there is a strong degree of genotypic-phenotypic correlation in inherited NF2, genetic testing is sometimes useful in people with this disorder.

Clinical Indications for Testing

Genetic tests are used most often to identify children who are at risk of inheriting NF2 because they are born into families with a history of the disorder. Once such a child is confirmed to have an *NF2* mutation, he or she can be monitored periodically for development of manifestations so that treatment can be administered at appropriate times. These tests have some limitations, however. Direct DNA tests that are currently available find mutations in ~65% of people tested.[5,6] Therefore, they are not completely accurate. As a result, even a child who tests negative for an *NF2* mutation should continue to be monitored until early adulthood to ensure that manifestations do not develop. Another caution is that the tests are not yet sensitive enough to predict phenotype. Linkage analysis is more accurate, providing that other family members agree to participate.

Availability

Although still difficult to access, genetic testing for NF2 is emerging. Clinical testing is available at a handful of sites throughout the world, including two in the United States. Only physicians may request such testing for a patient.

◆ Genetic Counseling

As was demonstrated in the previous chapter, the pathogenesis of NF1 and NF2 is quite complex and difficult for most patients and families to understand. For that reason, many people who have neurofibromatosis or have a child with the disorder will benefit from a genetic counseling session. Although specifics vary, the goal of genetic counseling is to translate complicated medical information in a way that a layperson can understand. The genetic counselor will then help the person with a genetic disorder (or the parents) understand the issues involved in various decisions, such as choosing among treatments or deciding whether to have a child. What a genetic counselor does not do is actually make those decisions; his or her role is to explain the risks and benefits and provide estimates of how likely it is that complications might occur.

A genetic counseling session usually involves a consultation with a physician, nurse, or specially trained genetic counselor. Primary care physicians are usually willing to make a referral to an appropriate counselor, or patients can contact professional societies.

Often the first step in a genetic counseling session is to confirm a diagnosis. To do so, the genetic counselor may review individual medical records, ask questions about family medical history, and review results from medical tests. He or she may also conduct a physical exam. The next step usually involves a discussion of what manifestations the disorder causes, how those manifestations develop, and what options exist for treatment. The counselor should also discuss how the disorder can be passed on to offspring. By the end of the session, the person seeking counseling should understand the genetic disorder better and feel more empowered to make decisions.

Receiving a diagnosis of NF1 or NF2 can be upsetting, especially if there is no family history of the condition and it is discovered incidentally. As a result, it's normal to feel confused, anxious, scared, and depressed. Patients should expect, and health care providers should be prepared, to spend time addressing emotional as well as medical concerns. Patient education brochures and other educational materials are helpful, as are referrals to support groups and patient advocacy organizations.

◆ The Personal Perspective

Nancy B.: "My twin sister and I look a lot alike, but we didn't know if we were identical. We actually found out through a clinical trial. This was probably 15 or 20 years ago, when I was 30, and we had genetic testing done. The test involves doing more and more refined DNA probes until either a difference is found or they give up. In our case, they did give up and we were told that there was a 99.9% chance that we are identical. The interesting thing is that even though my sister and I are identical, we have some of the same manifestations and some different ones. You'd like to think that there is a genotype-phenotype correlation, but that is not the case in NF1.

"I didn't get married until I was 37. I had already decided that I would not have any children, so that was of course something we discussed before getting married. Because NF is a dominant trait, there is a 50% chance that each of our children might have NF. More importantly, there is not a way to predict severity. I knew I couldn't live with myself if I had a child who was severely affected. I'd feel guilty about causing emotional and physical pain to an innocent child. So that was always a concern when I was dating. When I got serious about the man who is now my husband, I knew I had to get this out in the open. Everyone should be able to have a child without worries like these. Fortunately, not having children wasn't an issue for him, and we have been happily married for 13 years. Still, I often think about what it would be like to have children."

Kellie C.: "I knew there was a 50/50 chance that each of my children could inherit NF1. We basically put our faith in God. We came to the conclusion that no one is guaranteed a perfect pregnancy or a healthy child. We have two kids. David is 4 $^1/_2$ years old and Danielle is 19 months old. David definitely does not have NF1. Danielle has three or four café-au-lait spots, so we're watching her. Our primary care physician delivered both my children. And when I was pregnant, she said, 'Worse things can happen than NF1.' I think people need to remember that most cases of NF1 are mild. The chances are low that NF1 will be severe. I think you need to keep it in perspective."

Dolores G.: "My daughter Susan was diagnosed with NF1 in the early 1970s. The doctors did try to sit down and explain what NF was, but the information was all wrong. At that time the consensus was that NF had to be passed on by one of the parents. There was no talk of spontaneous mutations. My husband and I were both examined at the hospital. I have a lot of freckles, so therefore I was diagnosed with NF. As it turns out, I didn't have it. I was 'de-diagnosed' later, as I like to say.

"But at the time, they decided I had NF1 also, because of the freckles. We sat down with the head of the hospital. He was a personal friend and ex-boss of mine. And we talked about this. My husband and I both asked him, what do you think that we should do? We'd like to have more children. Even before we got married we said we would adopt as well as have biological children. But then I got pregnant with Susan, so our plans to adopt were postponed. He said that if he was in our position, since we already had two daughters, that he would probably not have other kids because the chance of having another child with NF1 was so high. And you only needed one parent to pass NF on."

Adam G.: "I know there's a 50% chance that I could pass this on to my children. I am concerned about it. One of my biggest faults is that I always think too far in the future. I consciously try not to think about this whole issue yet. It is a concern, but I try not to let it get to me right now. My mom says that by the time it's an issue, there may be a cure for NF2."

Martha L.: "My husband and I don't have children. As much as I love life, and kids, I decided I didn't want to put anyone through the life I have had to lead. My husband completely understood and knew before we got married how I felt about it. We don't have a history of NF in my family, so my parents didn't know that any of their children would have NF. I am the only one out of three that has it.

"When I got married at 24, I gave the world a deadline of my thirtieth birthday to find a cure or treatment for NF, and if that weren't available, I would give up my dream of having my own children. Unfortunately, no cure or treatment was found."

Tamra M.: "I've thought about children a lot. I talked it over with one of my teachers who was close to me. We were talking one day and she asked me whether I would have children, and I wasn't sure. A year later, I did a report on orphans and homeless children. I found out how many orphans there were. So I thought, there's the solution! I'm thinking I'll adopt children because there are so many who need homes."

Angela W.: "I knew I wanted to have children more than anything. We thought we'd wait a year or two after we got married. God kind of made the decision for us. We decided it was a blessing and God's will, so we were going to go ahead with it and let nature and fate decide what happens.

"We did talk with a genetic counselor when I was 5 or 6 months pregnant. It helped my husband more than it helped me. I knew a lot of the information already, but it was hard to explain to someone else. The counseling session helped my husband understand how NF1 can be inherited and that the pregnancy might worsen some of my symptoms.

"I think if you have NF1 and you're thinking of having kids, you need to be willing to accept whatever problems there might be. Know what you're getting into. So far my baby looks healthy and I'm happy with that. But if Davin has complications down the road, I have no regrets. I'm willing to accept whatever comes."

References

1. Ruggieri M, Huson SM. The clinical and diagnostic implications of mosaicism in the neurofibromatoses. Neurology 2001;56:1433–1443
2. Wu BL, Austin MA, Schneider GH, Boles RG, Korf BR. Deletion of the entire NF1 gene detected by FISH: four deletion patients associated with severe manifestations. Am J Med Genet 1995;59:528–535
3. Shen MH, Harper PS, Upadhyaya M. Molecular genetics of neurofibromatosis type 1 (NF1). J Med Genet 1996;33:2–17
4. Friedman JM, Gutmann DH, MacCollin M, Riccardi VM, eds. Neurofibromatosis: Phenotype, Natural History, and Pathogenesis. 3rd ed. Baltimore: Johns Hopkins University Press; 1999:102
5. MacCollin M, Ramesh V, Jacoby LB, et al. Mutational analysis of patients with neurofibromatosis 2. Am J Hum Genet 1994;55:314–320
6. Parry DM, MacCollin MM, Kaiser-Kupfer MI, et al. Germ-line mutations in the neurofibromatosis 2 gene: correlations with disease severity and retinal abnormalities. Am J Hum Genet 1996;59:529–539

5

Diagnosis and Overall Management of Neurofibromatosis 1

A diagnosis of neurofibromatosis 1 (NF1) can be unsettling and even frightening for the person who receives it. Fortunately, most people with NF1 will develop mild to moderate manifestations, and if complications arise they are generally not life threatening. Many people with NF1 lead happy and productive lives: they often marry, have children, and work in various careers. The challenge is to acknowledge the seriousness of the disorder, seek regular medical attention, and deal with complications as they arise.

The most common NF1 manifestations are café-au-lait spots, neurofibromas, Lisch nodules, and skinfold freckling, although additional manifestations of the disorder may appear. *Learning disabilities* are also common. Many people with NF1 tend to have larger-than-normal head circumference, and are shorter than average. Although people with NF1 are at somewhat increased risk of developing certain rare cancers of the brain, spinal cord, and nerves, their risk of other cancers is about the same as that of the general population.[1(p54)] Each of the typical manifestations of NF1 is described briefly in this chapter. Much greater detail about the features and complications is provided in Chapters 6 through 9.

◆ Diagnostic Criteria for Neurofibromatosis 1

The diagnostic criteria established for NF1 are outlined in Table **5–1**. A diagnosis of NF1 involves two possible scenarios. In the case of a child born to a parent who has NF1, diagnosis is generally straightforward, for one of the diagnostic criteria (a first-degree relative with the disorder) has already been met. If the child also has NF1, the first feature to appear is usually café-au-lait spots. Diagnosis of the inherited form of NF1 is therefore usually made in the first or second year of life. Skinfold freckling, the next most common skin feature of NF1, is usually visible by age 7.[2(p610)]

Diagnosis may be more of a challenge when a child suspected of having NF1 is born to parents without the disorder. Whenever a child is born with six or more café-au-lait spots, the most likely cause is NF1; familial café-au-lait spot syndrome is rare. However, it may take several years to confirm the diagnosis. In most cases, additional criteria emerge by the time the child is 8 years old.[2(p613)]

In most cases, physicians can diagnose NF1 by making a few modifications to a standard diagnostic workup to focus on the most common features of NF1. Follow-up care depends on what manifestations and complications develop. In general, the best approach to management of NF1 is to adopt a strategy of watchful waiting. This consists of anticipatory guidance (information about what types of manifestations are possible, when they might arise, and what tests might be necessary) and periodic

Table 5–1   Diagnostic Criteria for Neurofibromatosis 1 (NF1)

The patient should have two or more of the following:

1. Six or more café-au-lait spots:
  • 1.5 cm or larger in individuals past puberty
  • 0.5 cm or larger in individuals before puberty

2. Two or more neurofibromas of any type, or one or more plexiform neurofibromas
3. Freckling in the axilla or groin
4. Optic glioma (tumor of the optic pathway)
5. Two or more Lisch nodules (benign iris hamartomas)

6. A distinctive bony lesion:
  • Dysplasia (abnormal development) of the sphenoid bone
  • Dysplasia or thinning of long bone cortex

7. A first degree relative with NF1

Adapted from Gutmann DH, Aylsworth A, Carey JC, et al. The diagnostic evaluation and multidisciplinary management of neurofibromatosis 1 and neurofibromatosis 2. JAMA 1997;278:52, with permission.

surveillance for medical complications. For many people with NF1, annual follow-up visits are sufficient; more frequent visits may be necessary if complications develop.

If a pediatrician or internist makes the initial diagnosis, it is wise to consider a referral to an NF1 specialist or a neurofibromatosis clinic for follow-up. A list of neurofibromatosis clinics is provided at the NF Web site: *www.nf.org*. Most patients regularly see an NF1 specialist in addition to a general practitioner and specialists for any other medical conditions that may exist. Referral to specific specialists is appropriate in the following situations:

- Complications develop that affect the eyes, nervous system, or spine or bones.
- Discrete neurofibromas cause pain or disfigurement and require surgery.
- Plexiform neurofibromas interfere with normal body structure or organ functioning.
- Pain requires management.
- Malignancies develop.

◆ Natural History of Neurofibromatosis 1

The natural history of a disorder refers to its development and progression over time. In general, NF1 is a progressive disorder, which means that its features will become more numerous, and possibly more severe, with time. It is important to point out, however, that some people do not experience progression. They may have manifestations that seem to stay the same and do not change appreciably over time. Table **5–2** summarizes when typical features might present. Because NF1 is so variable, however, it is impossible to predict what course a given patient's disorder will take.

Mortality is often a concern for patients, because some research has suggested that people with NF1 have a shorter life span than people without the disorder. However, two population studies on the subject are fairly small, each involving 70 or 80 people with NF1, and at least one is based on old data.[3,4] The consensus now is that some people with NF1 die earlier than expected, mainly due to malignancies or complications from surgery. Such early deaths shift the average life expectancy curve for people with NF1 to the left, so that the average life span is less than that for people without the disorder. In most cases, however, individuals with NF1 can expect to live with their disorder for a normal life span. People with NF1 tend to die of the same causes as people without the disorder, such as heart disease and cancer.

Table 5–2   Neurofibromatosis 1 Features Through the Life Span

Congenital	• Café-au-lait spots (usually visible by age 1 or 2) • Plexiform neurofibromas (usually visible by age 1) • Tibial dysplasia (severe cases seen early; mild cases may take longer)
Ages 3 to 6	• Skinfold freckling (usually appears between 3 and 5) • Optic gliomas (most frequently occur between 4 and 6)
Ages 6 to 10	• Lisch nodules (occasionally appear earlier) • Learning disabilities • Short stature; large head (may be evident earlier) • Rapidly progressing scoliosis (between 6 and 10) • Hypertension (usually associated with renal artery stenosis, but may be caused by pheochromocytoma) • Migraine headaches or abdominal pain
Late childhood, early adolescence	• Dermal neurofibromas • Milder form of scoliosis • Precocious puberty
Adulthood	• Increase in size and number of neurofibromas • Pain • Malignant peripheral nerve sheath tumors • Hypertension (usually similar to that in the general population)

◆ Guidelines for Initial Evaluation and Follow-Up Visits

An initial evaluation of someone suspected of having NF1, and routine follow-up visits, are quite similar. The consultation should focus on common manifestations and features associated with NF1, and also include an evaluation of less common, yet potentially more serious, complications of the disorder.[1(pp52–54)] An overview of a comprehensive evaluation is listed in Table **5–3**, and explained in further detail in this chapter and those that follow.

Medical History

A review of a person's medical history should include greater attention to features of NF1 as well as a more general assessment of overall health and any other medical concerns. Because many features of NF1 are age-dependent, it is important to determine when the patient's manifestations first appeared. Whenever possible, the patient should bring, and the doctor should review, medical records. These are helpful in establishing a timeline as well as providing valuable medical information. A thorough

Table 5–3   Initial Diagnostic Assessment for Neurofibromatosis 1

Medical history focusing on manifestations of NF1:

- Pigmented skin lesions
- Dermal tumors
- Learning disabilities
- Vision problems
- Seizures
- Headaches
- Scoliosis
- Orthopedic abnormalities
- Hypertension
- Review of previous medical reports

Physical examination:

- Measurement of height, weight, and head circumference
- Measurement of blood pressure
- Examination of skin for café-au-lait spots, skinfold freckling, and dermal tumors
- Inspection of long bones for abnormalities, especially bowing of the tibia
- Examination of the back for scoliosis
- Age-appropriate neurological examination, including assessment of limbs for weakness and of eyes for *proptosis* (bulging of the eye) or *strabismus* (problems focusing one eye in conjunction with the other)

Ophthalmological examination:

- Complete examination to detect optic glioma
- Slit-lamp examination to detect Lisch nodules

Evaluation of family members:

- Family history for signs and symptoms of NF1
- Full assessment of any relative reported or suspected to have NF1
- Full assessment of both parents and all children of someone with NF1

Laboratory and imaging studies:

- Ordered only to evaluate complications suspected because of the medical history, physical examination, or ophthalmological examination

Adapted from Friedman JM. Evaluation and management. In: Friedman JM, Gutmann DH, MacCollin M, Riccardi VM, eds. Neurofibromatosis: Phenotype, Natural History, and Pathogenesis. 3rd ed. Baltimore: Johns Hopkins University Press; 1999:93, with permission.

medical history to diagnose NF1 should cover the following areas. During follow-up visits, any relevant issues should be revisited, to determine if anything has changed since the last visit.

Skin

Because the skin manifestations of NF1 appear at different times in life, the questions asked will depend on the age of the patient. The point is to determine whether the patient is aware of having any café-au-lait spots, skinfold freckling, or neurofibromas.

Vision

Questions about whether a child has had any vision changes help to determine whether the optic nerve is functioning properly, and whether the child might have an optic glioma.

Learning Problems

Asking about a child's school performance is important because difficulty with schoolwork may indicate an underlying learning disability. Learning disabilities are found in half of all children with NF1 and are the most common complications of the disorder in childhood.[5] If a learning disability is suspected, referral should be made for a thorough assessment and support facilities (see Chapter 8).

Skeletal Abnormalities

Skeletal abnormalities, ranging from an abnormal shape of the eye socket *(sphenoid dysplasia)* to a bowing of the lower leg *(tibial dysplasia),* are *congenital* and so are usually apparent in childhood. Patients and families are usually aware of any obvious abnormalities. *Scoliosis,* on the other hand, may be so mild that they will not know about it.

Headaches or Seizures

Because NF1 engages the central nervous system, some people with the disorder experience headaches and even *epilepsy*. The type of headaches and epileptic *seizures* experienced by people with NF1 are indistinguishable from those experienced by people without the disorder, but some studies suggest they may occur more frequently in NF1.

Family Medical History

Because NF1 is inherited in about half of all cases, the medical history of close relatives is relevant when making a diagnosis. One diagnostic criterion is having a first-degree relative with the disorder: a parent, sibling, or child. Because milder forms of NF1 may never have been diagnosed, however, it is also important to ask about second-degree relatives: grandparents, aunts, uncles, and cousins, and even their descendants. If NF1 is suspected in any of the patient's first- and second-degree relatives, it is important that a diagnosis be confirmed through medical records and, if possible, physical examination of these relatives.

Physical Examination

An initial evaluation for NF1 involves careful attention to the skin, because dermal manifestations of the disorder develop early and are most often used to establish diagnosis. Skeletal and neurological health should also be assessed, inasmuch as both systems may be involved in NF1. Initial and routine follow-up examinations should include a systematic assessment to detect any other complications of NF1.

Because many of the features of NF1 are age dependent, physicians and patients alike should become familiar with what manifestations are likely to be revealed at different stages of life. Not everyone with NF1 will experience every feature, and sometimes features develop in someone earlier or later than expected (see Table 5–2).

Growth Measurements

Annual height, weight, and head circumference measurements are important and should be compared with standard growth charts. Large head circumference is common in NF1 and can be used to aid diagnosis, but it does not cause medical consequences. Accelerated growth in height or weight, however, is one of the first signs of *precocious puberty*, a complication of NF1 that can result when an optic glioma develops in the optic chiasm.

Blood Pressure

Blood pressure should be measured, even in children. Although high blood pressure (known medically as *hypertension*) can arise in anyone, in people with NF1 it may develop because of two rare complications of the disorder. They are renal artery stenosis, blockage of the artery leading to the kidney, and pheochromocytoma, a rare and usually benign adrenal gland tumor. Hypertension in children, and persistent hypertension in adults that does not respond to standard blood pressure medications, should therefore be carefully evaluated (see Chapter 9).

Skin Features

Dermal manifestations of NF1 can develop anywhere; the patient should disrobe so that the skin can be examined thoroughly. Occasionally café-au-lait spots and freckling will be close in color to surrounding skin and will be detected only through careful examination.

◆ **Café-Au-Lait Spots** Six or more café-au-lait spots (Fig. **5–1**), areas of pigmentation darker in color than surrounding skin, are one of the hallmark

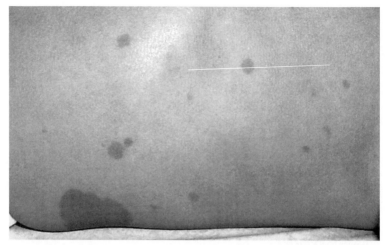

Figure 5–1   Café-au-lait spots are areas of pigmentation darker in color than surrounding skin. There is no correlation between the number or size of café-au-lait spots and the number or severity of other NF1 manifestations a person will experience.

signs of NF1. Although these areas of pigmentation cause no medical effects, they are extremely useful in making a diagnosis. There is no correlation between the number or size of café-au-lait spots and the number or severity of other NF1 manifestations a person will experience. Less than 1% of children *without* NF1 who are under the age of 5 have more than two café-au-lait spots[6]; hence, multiple spots are usually an indication that a child has the disorder. Only 10% of unaffected adults have even one café-au-lait spot that is 1.5 cm or larger, though 90% of adults with NF1 do.[7]

Café-au-lait spots are sometimes visible at birth, but if they are not, they will generally appear by the time the child is 1 or 2 years old.[1(p53)] Although some café-au-lait spots are big enough to be obvious, smaller ones can be distinguished from ordinary freckles by their size. In a child who has not yet entered puberty, six or more spots that are 0.5 cm (5 mm, about one-fifth of an inch) or larger meet the diagnostic criteria for NF1. Past puberty, spots 1.5 cm (15 mm, about one-half of an inch) or larger meet the criteria. Measurements should be taken at the widest diameter.

Café-au-lait spots may vary in size and number. In adults, they are usually between 10 and 30 mm in diameter.[8(pp37,40)] Sometimes they are so small that they resemble freckles, or so large that they cover an entire part of the body on one side, especially when located on the trunk and buttocks. Most café-au-lait spots seen in NF1 are oval in shape, with well-defined borders. Sometimes, however, they have different shapes, ragged borders, or are pale in color and poorly defined. They can originate almost anywhere on the body, but those associated with NF1 usually are not found on the scalp, eyebrows, palms, or soles. Café-au-lait spots "grow" with a child, becoming progressively larger with age until adulthood. Additional spots may also become visible with time, although it is likely they were there all along and became darker with sun exposure.

The spots tend to be of uniform color, although pigment variations do exist. In light-skinned people, they are tan, whereas in darker skinned people they may be dark brown or black. In people with fair skin, the spots may be so light that they are hard to distinguish from surrounding skin.

Two-toned café-au-lait spots (a darker area located within a lighter one) probably result from a small café-au-lait spot developing within a larger café-au-lait spot. Typically café-au-lait spots darken in color when exposed to sun; thus as the skin tans, the spots remain clearly visible. A scar within a café-au-lait spot, however, will have less pigmentation than the rest of the spot and may resemble surrounding skin. Occasionally a café-au-lait spot is surrounded by lighter skin, producing a halo-like effect. This probably indicates that a café-au-lait spot is located within another area of pigmentation, not related to NF1, known as a Mongolian spot.

◆ **Skinfold Freckling**   Skinfold freckles (Fig. **5–2**) are areas of pigmentation similar in color to café-au-lait spots but smaller in diameter. Such

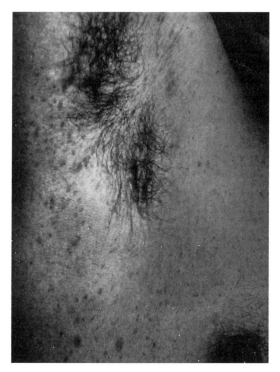

Figure 5–2   Axillary freckles are smaller versions of café-au-lait spots. They can be differentiated from sun-induced freckles primarily on the basis of location.

freckles tend to develop where skinfolds form naturally or as a result of weight gain. The most common areas where they are found are under the arms (axillary freckling), in the groin area (inguinal freckling), the underside of breasts, upper eyelids, and base of the neck.

Because skinfold freckling is the second most frequent age-dependent manifestation of NF1, evident in ~9 in 10 people with NF1, it is extremely useful in establishing a diagnosis.[1(p52)] When a child is suspected of having NF1 because he or she has multiple café-au-lait spots, skinfold freckling provides a reliable way to confirm an early diagnosis. Such freckling most often first appears when a child is between 3 and 5 years old.[9] By middle age, 89% of people with NF1 have axillary freckling, and 56% have inguinal freckling.[10]

Skinfold freckles associated with NF1 tend to be 1 to 3 mm in diameter, and can be distinguished from ordinary freckles mainly by location: they are usually arranged in clusters in areas of the body not exposed to the sun. Groin freckling is usually noted first; sometimes it is visible at birth, but more often it is observed in early childhood. Skinfold freckles on other areas of the body may become noticeable later in childhood and into adulthood.

The freckles seen in NF1 probably develop because the low levels of neurofibromin have an effect on how the skin functions and may make it more vulnerable to changes induced by environmental factors. Physical characteristics of skinfolds somehow modify the expression of neurofibromin. Possible environmental factors that come into play include an absence of light, warmth, moisture, and normal skin secretions such as salt. Friction may also contribute to the development of NF1 freckles, considering that they are often seen along the collar line or where a brassiere rubs against the skin.

◆ **Generalized Increased Pigmentation**   Some people with NF1 develop more generalized increased skin pigmentation as they grow older, which results in an overall darker cast to their skin. It is not known why this occurs, for the phenomenon has not been studied very carefully. The condition may cause psychological distress but has no serious medical ramifications.

Neurofibromas

The tumors that are another hallmark sign of NF1 may grow anywhere on or in the body, usually starting just before puberty and continuing through adulthood into old age (see Chapter 6). Cutaneous or dermal neurofibromas are those on the surface of the skin (the epidermis). They may at first resemble mosquito bites that don't heal: small dome-shaped

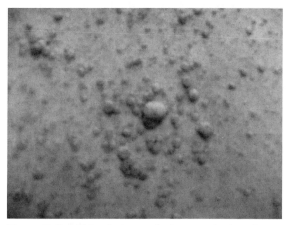

Figure 5–3 This photograph shows a cluster of neurofibromas on the skin (moderate severity).

bumps that are soft and fleshy to the touch. Subcutaneous neurofibromas are those located within the two bottom layers of the skin (the dermis and hypodermis), or just under the skin. They may create a slight protuberance or may cause the skin to look dappled in certain lights.

Some people with NF1 develop only a few neurofibromas; others develop thousands (Figs. **5–3** and **5–4**). They can develop anywhere on or in the body, including nipples and genitalia. The number and location of

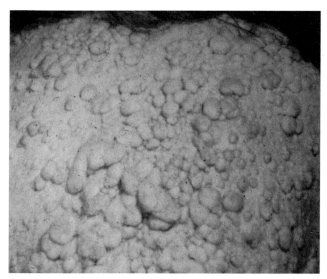

Figure 5–4 This 35-year-old woman has many neurofibromas on the trunk of her body—an unusually severe manifestation of these tumors.

neurofibromas has no correlation with the severity of other NF1 manifestations, but as a hallmark feature of the disorder these benign tumors are useful in diagnosis. They may also become a chief source of anxiety for patients, who are understandably worried about the impact of these tumors on their appearance and comfort. Fortunately, most people with NF1 do not become disfigured. Although there is currently no way to prevent neurofibromas from developing, options for management do exist (see Chapter 6).

◆ **Plexiform Neurofibromas**   These occur in NF1 in about one in three peoplc,[10] although these tumors may never cause symptoms. *Plexiform neurofibromas* are usually congenital, although they may go undetected for years if they are not visible or causing any discomfort. Most are diffuse, growing along the length of a nerve or even engulfing several nerve shafts. These may be visible in some infants and young children as a large patch of skin that is darker in color than surrounding skin, or as an area of skin that appears thick or swollen (Fig. **5–5**). Location and size vary. Upon *palpation*, a diffuse plexiform neurofibroma feels soft and malleable.

Some diffuse plexiform neurofibromas grow so large that they cause disfigurement and may even interfere with normal bone growth and development and even function. Diffuse plexiform neurofibromas that grow on the face or neck generally develop in the first year of life; those that develop in other parts of the body may appear any time in childhood but rarely after puberty.[11]

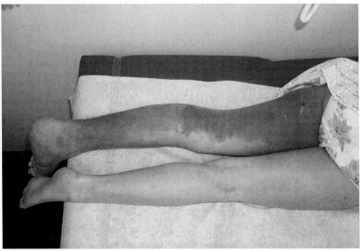

Figure 5–5   The hyperpigmentation in an area of skin on this child's leg indicates the presence of a plexiform neurofibroma along the sciatic nerve.

Less common are discrete nodular plexiform neurofibromas that originate from a single site on a nerve. These are usually less easily detected in childhood. Although nodular plexiform neurofibromas may not cause any symptoms, in general they are more likely to become painful than are diffuse plexiform neurofibromas (see Chapter 6).

In 5[8(p152)] to 10%[12] of people with NF1, neurofibromas may become malignant, transforming into malignant peripheral nerve sheath tumors (MPNSTs). This rarely if ever happens to dermal neurofibromas; malignant transformation most often occurs in preexisting plexiform neurofibromas. The first sign of such transformation is usually chronic pain. The tumor may also feel hard or firm, rather than soft, when palpated. This is a potentially fatal complication of NF1 and should be thoroughly evaluated whenever it is suspected.

Inspection of Bones and Spine

NF1 is associated with several bone malformations that are not only important in establishing diagnosis, but also may require medical attention (see Chapter 9). Although less frequent than skin features of NF1, such bone manifestations tend to be more serious. A physical examination, therefore, should include an assessment to detect any bone abnormalities. In young children, early detection of such abnormalities provides time to intervene so that serious complications, such as disfigurement, fractures, or *pseudoarthrosis*, can be avoided.

The long bone most often vulnerable is the tibia, the larger of the two bones in the shin, below the knee. In severe cases of dysplasia, the leg will become bowed as the child grows and places weight on the legs. Less severe cases may require close inspection of both legs, to see if they are asymmetrical; the shin of one leg may also have a protrusion the other does not. Facial asymmetry associated with the eyes and forehead may be caused by defects in the sphenoid bone of the skull.

In people who have NF1, scoliosis is found in about one in 10.[8(p262)] The most common type seen involves a long, gently curved C-shaped malformation involving much of the spine (usually about eight to 10 *vertebrae*). This is similar to the type of scoliosis that is present in the general population, but it tends to occur a few years earlier in children with NF1—generally in late childhood or early adolescence. This mild type of scoliosis can be diagnosed by asking the patient to bend forward at the waist; any extra fullness or bulging seen on one side of the back or the other may indicate curvature in the spine (Fig. **5–6**). An x-ray of the spine will then provide additional information on the nature of the curve and how aggressively it should be treated.

Far less common, and more serious, is a type of spinal curvature known as dystrophic scoliosis. This type of scoliosis creates a sharp,

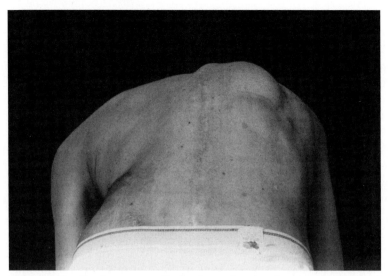

Figure 5–6   To diagnose scoliosis, the patient is asked to bend forward while the examiner looks for increased fullness on either side of the trunk.

almost angular curve and generally encompasses only a limited portion of the spine (five vertebrae or fewer). This is an earlier onset, rapidly progressing form of scoliosis that requires more aggressive management. If this type of scoliosis is going to develop in a child, it will usually occur between 6 and 10 years of age.[8(p263)] Because this form of scoliosis is associated only with NF1, it can be used to establish diagnosis.

Neurological Assessment

To determine if there are neurological impairments, it is important to test the patient's reflexes and make other assessments of neurological functioning. The exact tests selected will depend on the patient's age. Reflexes that are minimal or absent (areflexia) or weakness of the arms or legs (leading to falls at home, for instance) may indicate that neurofibromas in the spine are interfering with normal function.

Ophthalmological Examination

If a child is diagnosed with NF1, or suspected of having the disorder, he or she should undergo regular annual ophthalmological exams until the peak risk of developing an optic glioma has passed, generally accepted as age 7. Although the National Institutes of Health (NIH) Consensus Committee recommended that annual ophthalmological testing continue until age 10, and then periodically afterward,[1(p53)] there are no firm guidelines on this issue and many physicians recommend that testing be relaxed earlier. Features associated with NF1 include the following:

Lisch Nodules

These small, dome-shaped bumps on the iris (Fig. **5–7**), the colored part of the eye that surrounds the pupil, are the most common eye manifestation of NF1. Lisch nodules eventually are visible in almost all people with the disorder, and are second only to skin manifestations in terms of establishing a diagnosis. These distinctive nodules are named for Karl Lisch,[13] an Austrian ophthalmologist who in 1937 first associated them with the disorder that would later become known as NF1. Lisch nodules do not interfere with vision and are not associated with other eye tumors. Their presence or absence is in no way associated with severity of other NF1 features.

Typically Lisch nodules first appear when a child is 5 years old.[14] By age 6 in children with NF1, 15 to 20% will have Lisch nodules on one or both irises[15]; by adulthood, 95% of people with the disorder have Lisch nodules.[15-18]

Only an experienced ophthalmologist can distinguish Lisch nodules from ordinary iris freckles or other conditions that can cause similar bumps or discoloration in the iris. To determine whether someone has Lisch nodules, the ophthalmologist must perform an examination with a *slit lamp*, an illuminated microscope. Viewed with a slit lamp, Lisch

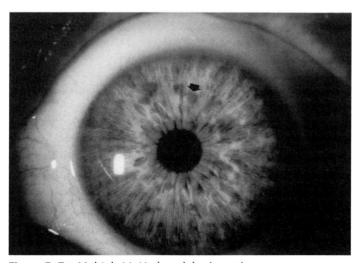

Figure 5–7   Multiple iris Lisch nodules (arrow).

nodules are revealed as three-dimensional translucent nodules on the iris. Lisch nodules may be tan or glassy in color. They may be darker than the iris if it is blue, hazel, or light brown, or lighter than the iris if it is medium or dark brown.

Lisch nodules tend to develop in equal numbers on both eyes. In young children, however, only one or two may be visible at first.[16] It is not known why Lisch nodules develop in people with NF1, although, like other features relating to pigmentation, Lisch nodules develop from tissue that originates in the neural crest stage of embryonic development.

Optic Gliomas

These malignant, but generally low-grade, tumors can develop anywhere along the optic nerve and usually occur in early childhood, whether a child has NF1 or not. Depending on their location, *optic gliomas* can cause significant problems such as loss of vision or early puberty. If an optic glioma is going to cause symptoms, this will usually occur by the time a child is 6 years old.[19,20] In most cases, an optic glioma is diagnosed by the time a child is 3 years old.[2(613)] If a child has an optic glioma, it is a reliable sign that he or she may have NF1.

A thorough ophthalmological exam, described in detail in Chapter 7, is required to determine whether a child has an optic glioma. Most children diagnosed with optic gliomas first experience visual defects such as optic nerve atrophy, swelling of the optic nerve *(papilledema)*, abnormal focusing of the eyes together *(strabismus)*, or defects in color vision. Bulging of the eye *(proptosis)* may indicate the presence of a tumor. The child may sustain a loss of visual acuity, with no other symptoms.[8(p209)] If the optic glioma develops in the optic chiasm, the child may experience precocious puberty. It is important to monitor height and weight measurements of children diagnosed with or suspected of having NF1, and to compare them to standard growth charts. Accelerated growth is one of the first signs of precocious puberty.

Additional Testing

Any further testing should be done only when clinically indicated by physical findings or reported symptoms. Periodic routine screening is of little to no value, because it will not shape management of NF1. Typical tests, and the situations under which they are warranted, are listed below.

Genetic Testing

As discussed in Chapter 4, in most cases genetic tests for NF1 are not necessary to establish a diagnosis.

Magnetic Resonance Imaging (MRI) Scans

An MRI scan of one location in the body may be necessary to detect a tumor such as an optic glioma, or to determine whether a plexiform neurofibroma is causing a particular symptom.

Far more controversial is the use of baseline and other routine MRI brain scans in children. T2-weighted MRI brain scans of children with NF1 sometimes reveal unidentified bright objects (UBOs), which are isolated areas of signal hyperintensity on the developed image. Although UBOs occur in about six of 10 children with NF1, they do not seem to have any clinical significance.[11] There is some evidence that UBOs are correlated with cognitive deficits, although the fact that a child has UBOs does not mean he or she will have such deficits. UBOs are not correlated with brain tumors or other manifestations of NF1. They also tend to disappear as the child grows into adulthood.

Some physicians argue that, besides detecting UBOs, baseline and other routine MRI scans are useful in confirming a diagnosis in some children who do not yet have features matching the diagnostic criteria, or help to identify complications before they cause symptoms. Opponents counter that MRI scans are costly and require sedation of children, with the attendant risks. The scans are not sensitive enough to guide management decisions, yet may raise anxiety when they reveal something in the brain such as a UBO or some other finding of unknown significance. Although there are different views on this topic, the current expert consensus is that, in most cases, baseline and other routine MRI brain scans are not necessary, and that management should be guided by symptoms.

X-Rays

X-rays of the skull, spine, or limbs are appropriate if a bone malformation is suspected, or if the patient is experiencing pain or other symptoms. X-rays of the chest will detect any internal tumors that are compressing the airway or otherwise may be significant.

Electroencephalograms (EEGs)

The electroencephalogram (EEG), a test that examines electrical activity of the brain, may be necessary if the patient is experiencing seizures or other neurological difficulties.

Intelligence Quotient (IQ) and Psychological Testing

If a child is suspected of having an NF1-related learning disability, he or she should undergo a thorough evaluation. This should include an IQ test to assess intelligence, as well as a range of other tests to evaluate skills such as verbal and spatial abilities. Because children with NF1 may also exhibit certain behavioral patterns, such as hyperactivity and attention deficits, psychological testing may also be necessary (see Chapter 8).

◆ Differential Diagnosis: Distinguishing NF1 from Similar Conditions

In most cases it is possible to definitely determine whether someone has NF1 or not by using the consensus diagnostic criteria reviewed in this chapter. When there is any doubt, however, a physician may go through a process known as differential diagnosis. The physician reviews conditions that cause manifestations similar to NF1 to determine whether any of them may be causing the observed clinical features and symptoms. The alternate diagnoses most often considered during differential diagnosis for NF1 are reviewed briefly below.

Segmental NF1

Several subtypes for NF1 have been proposed over the years, but consensus exists about only one: *segmental* (or *mosaic*) NF1. Other proposed subtypes probably represent different variations of NF1, because the disorder causes so many types of manifestations and their severity can vary widely. Still other proposed subtypes are probably entirely different disorders that have features in common with NF1.

Segmental NF1 is a subtype of the disorder that occurs when the *NF1* gene is mutated sometime after the zygote (the fertilized cell) is formed at conception (see Mosaicism in Neurofibromatosis 1 and Neurofibromatosis 2 in Chapter 4). This form of the disorder may also be referred to as mosaic NF1, because features are restricted to distinct areas, almost like pieces of a mosaic. The person will develop café-au-lait spots, skinfold freckling, and neurofibromas in only one area of the body, such as a shoulder and arm, or in a leg.

The size of the area where signs of NF1 are found probably depends on how long after conception the *NF1* gene mutation occurs. The earlier it occurs in embryonic development, the greater the area of the body eventually involved. If the mutation occurs early enough in postzygotic development, a case of segmental NF1 may extend to so much of the body that it will be mistaken for a mild case of generalized NF1. In other cases, the mutation may occur so late in development that the person will develop only isolated features of the disorder, such as a few café-au-lait spots, or one or two dermal neurofibromas. Preliminary evidence indicates that segmental NF1 may also sometimes develop when there is a defect in genetic replication or repair, resulting in multiple individual cells harboring independent mutations in the *NF1* gene (see Chapter 4). The research in this area continues.

Segmental NF1 can be distinguished from generalized NF1 by determining what parts of the body are affected. Segmental NF1 is often confined to one side of the body, without crossing the midline that divides the body into right and left halves that are almost mirror images of one another. Generalized NF1, on the other hand, causes skin features and other manifestations to materialize at random anywhere on or in the body. In many cases, segmental NF1 can be diagnosed by adolescence, provided that multiple café-au-lait spots, neurofibromas, or other common features of NF1 develop at the expected age but are present in only a well-defined area of the body. Some people with segmental NF1 may experience such mild manifestations, however, that the disorder is never diagnosed. Or it may be diagnosed only in the event of a rare complication such as pain caused when a previously undetected subcutaneous neurofibroma presses on a nerve root.

Because segmental NF1 most often has its origins in a postzygotic genetic mutation, it is generally not inherited and does not develop in people with a family history of NF1. The exception, noted above, would be a defect in the genetic replication or repair mechanism, which could be inherited and could result in the mutation of the *NF1* gene as well as other genes. This quite likely occurs only very rarely. As discussed in Chapter 4, however, there is no way of knowing whether the eggs or sperm of a person diagnosed with segmental NF1 contain the mutation. It is therefore possible that a person with segmental NF1 can give birth to a child with generalized NF1.

Disorders with Skin Features Similar to NF1

Familial Café-Au-Lait Spots

Although it occurs only rarely, some families pass multiple café-au-lait spots from one generation to the next in autosomal dominant fashion, but they display no other characteristics similar to NF1. If a child has multiple café-au-lait spots, with no other features of NF1, it is important to ask the parents whether they have such spots (and examine them, if there is any question), to establish a diagnosis. The familial café-au-lait spot syndrome is so rare that in most cases it is safe to assume that a child with six or more café-au-lait spots greater than 5 mm in size does indeed have NF1, but has not yet developed additional features of the disorder. The child should undergo a comprehensive ophthalmological exam and be followed until an NF1 diagnosis can be confirmed or ruled out. Generally this takes several years, although in some cases children must be followed into adolescence.

LEOPARD Syndrome

Multiple dark spots, typically located on the neck and trunk (although they can occur anywhere), may indicate that a person has LEOPARD syndrome (lentigines, electrocardiographic abnormalities, ocular abnormalities, pulmonary stenosis, abnormal genitalia, retardation of growth, and deafness). This autosomal dominant disorder can be distinguished from NF1 in several ways. The spots in LEOPARD syndrome are benign skin lesions (lentigines) rather than areas of pigmentation. They are usually darker than café-au-lait spots. People with LEOPARD syndrome, as the above definition indicates, also may experience features not associated with NF1, such as mild-to-moderate deafness, pulmonary stenosis (a restriction of the area between the pulmonary artery and the right ventricle of the heart), and hypertrophic cardiomyopathy (a thickening of the heart muscle). Common features of NF1, such as dermal neurofibromas and Lisch nodules, do not develop in people with LEOPARD syndrome.

McCune-Albright Syndrome

People with this disorder may have multiple café-au-lait spots that are difficult to distinguish from those seen in NF1 (Fig. **5–8**). People with McCune-Albright syndrome, however, do not have common features of NF1 such as dermal neurofibromas, skinfold freckling, and Lisch nodules. At the same time, bone abnormalities tend to be more severe than those associated with NF1. People with McCune-Albright syndrome most often have polyostotic fibrous dysplasia, a condition in which fibrous tissue replaces bone marrow in several bones.

Disorders with Tumor Growth and Other Features Similar to NF1

Bannayan-Riley-Ruvalcaba Syndrome

People with this syndrome may have multiple subcutaneous tumors, café-au-lait spots, and large heads—all of which are features of NF1. However, a close examination of the subcutaneous tumors reveals that they are not neurofibromas, but either lipomas (benign tumors composed of fatty tissue) or hemangiomas (benign tumors composed of blood vessels). Café-au-lait spots may be present in Bannayan-Riley-Ruvalcaba syndrome, but are less numerous than those typical of NF1. People with this syndrome

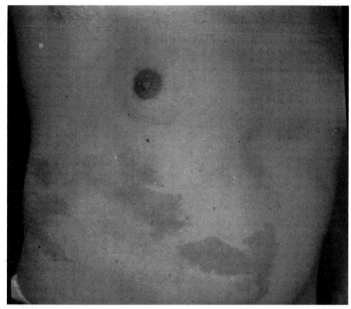

Figure 5–8 McCune-Albright syndrome. Note large café-au-lait spots occurring in a 6-year-old boy with bone cysts. There was no precocious puberty.

also have characteristics that are not usually seen in NF1, including mental retardation and spotted pigmentation on the penis.

Juvenile Hyaline Fibromatosis

This disorder involves a defect in the way that collagen is produced and broken down. Because collagen is a protein component of bone, skin, cartilage, and connective tissue, the defect may cause any one of several manifestations. Juvenile hyaline fibromatosis is sometimes mistaken for NF1 because it causes multiple benign subcutaneous tumors that can resemble neurofibromas. However, as the disorder progresses, it causes manifestations not usually seen in people with NF1, such as gums that become abnormally thick, and joints that become painful.

Congenital General Fibromatosis

This congenital disorder can cause tumor growth throughout the body by the time a child is 2 years old. Tumors may form on the skin, or be associated with muscles, bones, and organs in the abdomen. Unlike neurofibromas, however, the tumors that characterize congenital general fibromatosis do not continue to grow with age; instead, they are likely to regress and even disappear on their own.

Multiple Endocrine Neoplasia Type 2B

People with multiple endocrine neoplasia type 2B (MEN2B) sometimes develop neurofibromas and have multiple café-au-lait spots, and therefore may be misdiagnosed with NF1. More commonly, people with MEN2B develop various types of tumors involving the endocrine system, including pheochromocytoma, which is infrequently seen in NF1. People with MEN2B also exhibit skeletal features not associated with NF1, such as elongated limbs and other features more typical of Marfan's syndrome.

Multiple Lipomatosis

This rare inherited disorder is characterized by multiple benign skin tumors that resemble and feel like the dermal neurofibromas seen in NF1. A *biopsy*, however, will reveal that the tumors are lipomas, made up of fat cells. People with multiple lipomatosis tend to develop skin tumors on their arms and legs, but not on the shoulders and neck. There are no other features similar to those seen in NF1.

Noonan Syndrome

People with Noonan syndrome generally are short, have distinctive facial features (such as eyelids that droop and slant down, and incomplete development of the cheekbones), a broad neck, a concave chest, and congenital heart disorder. Although Noonan syndrome is distinct from NF1, there have been isolated cases in which both disorders have been found in the same person. The disorders have also been confused because some people with NF1 have facial features and other characteristics similar to those seen in Noonan syndrome.

Multiple Intradermal Nevi

Intradermal nevi are relatively common moles that can be skin colored or evenly pigmented. Although they can be flat, they usually are dome-shaped and round, and therefore may resemble neurofibromas. Intradermal nevi usually intrude only on the head, neck, or hands of adults, whereas neurofibromas can range over the entire body starting in adolescence. A person with multiple intradermal nevi will not have multiple café-au-lait spots or other common features of NF1.

Klippel-Trenaunay Syndrome

This is a rare congenital disorder in which a child is born with reddish-purple birthmarks (port-wine stains) and hemangiomas, masses of blood vessels that may protrude from the skin. People with this syndrome may also develop varicose veins, or experience excessive growth of soft tissue and bone in arms or legs. These features usually originate on only one side of the body.

Proteus Syndrome

This newly recognized syndrome was probably the disorder exhibited by Joseph Merrick, the so-called Elephant Man (see Chapter 1). Proteus syndrome does not imperil nerve tissue, however; instead, it may cause bone and soft tissue to grow excessively, usually on one side of the body, resulting in significant deformity. Especially the hands and feet may become enlarged, misshapen, and have skin that takes on a cauliflower appearance.

◆ The Personal Perspective

Nancy B: "It's kind of interesting how I found out. I was born in 1952. During my childhood, I don't think any one knew much about neurofibromatosis. My pediatrician noticed that I had many café-au-lait spots, as did my twin sister. Back then they were called birthmarks. But there was no medical condition associated with them, and because they didn't cause any problems, there was no need to discuss possible medical treatment. When I was about 18, I went to an endocrinologist because my menstrual cycle was so irregular, and he was the one who said he was quite sure I had neurofibromatosis. With NF1, you can have a very early or late onset of your menstrual cycle; that is what suggested to the endocrinologist that I had it.

"I don't see an NF specialist except when I have medical issues that could be related to it, which isn't very often. I do go to a gynecologist every year and get an annual mammogram, for I am at high risk for breast cancer. I recently saw a primary care physician because I hadn't had a regular checkup in several years. She suggested I see a dermatologist, a good idea even if you don't have NF1! The dermatologist was actually more concerned that I be followed regularly by a neurologist because of the NF1. I haven't done so yet."

Porter C.: "I was diagnosed with NF1 at age 12 in 1938. The doctor told my parents that the outcome was unpredictable and to 'treat her as if there were nothing wrong.' So I climbed trees, walked fences, and did what other kids did. I had café-au-lait spots and a lot of pain. My mother said that as an infant I cried for 2 weeks—cause unknown. I think, now, it was the tumors."

Diane D.: "Julie was born two weeks early. I knew something was different about her right from the start. I call it mother's intuition. I remember looking at her when she was only 6 weeks old, and she had an oddly shaped forehead and a droopy eye. Later on, we found out this was sphenoid dysplasia.

"At the time, I was going to a group pediatrics practice and I met with a different doctor each time. By the time Julie was 9 months old, she had developed multiple café-au-lait spots and I had a list of things I was concerned about. The last pediatrician I saw reviewed the list, examined Julie, and stepped out of the room briefly. When she came back, she said, 'I've made an appointment with the neurologist.' She knew.

"The pediatric neurologist ordered an MRI and did an assessment. When he met with us, he was using all sorts of long medical terms and told us he did not know about the prognosis. I immediately got on the computer and did research. Of course, some of what I found was frightening. I cried. Fortunately, I found the NF Foundation right away. I called them and they sent me a packet of information. I did some more research and found a specialist in Boston. We now have a team of specialists as well as our local pediatrician."

Dolores G.: "When Susan was born she had what the doctor called 'birthmarks'—a huge one covering her left knee, and one on her buttocks. Now we know they were café-au-lait spots, but at the time the doctor thought they were birthmarks.

"As a newborn, Susan was in a lot of distress. She cried and cried. We thought she was colicky. Then when Susan was about 16 months old, she developed what I assumed was a very severe UTI (urinary tract infection). She was almost potty trained and had gone to the bathroom to urinate, but then she started crying. When I looked, the whole toilet bowl was red.

"I called my pediatrician and said, 'I think we're dealing with an acute UTI.' He put her in the hospital and started doing tests. They did some tests and decided that there was some type of mass that was blocking her ureter. While we were in the hospital, the resident urologist came in and saw her, and then talked to my husband and me. He just nonchalantly said to us, 'Oh, your daughter has neurofibromatosis.' I had never heard of NF before. He just sort of dumped it on us and I think that he mentioned that you can develop tumors and that it can be life threatening. At that point, I kicked him out of the room."

Tamra M.: "I was diagnosed with NF1 when I was 7 months old. I had a small lump underneath the skin on my neck and café-au-lait spots. I don't remember when my parents told me, but I knew I had it when I was young. For as long as I can remember, I knew I had NF1. I'm the first person in my family to have it.

"I see a specialist at a children's hospital. My main doctor is a craniofacial surgeon. He's nice; he's really funny. About 2 years ago, I started seeing another doctor, a bone surgeon, for my spine. He's really nice too."

Angela W.: "I found out I had NF1 when I was about 13, when I started asking questions about why I had to go to the doctor every year and why I had café-au-lait spots. I was diagnosed at 6 at a children's hospital. My parents decided to wait to tell me until I started asking a lot of questions."

References

1. Gutmann DH, Aylsworth A, Carey JC, et al. The diagnostic evaluation and multidisciplinary management of neurofibromatosis 1 and neurofibromatosis 2. JAMA 1997;278:51–57
2. DeBella K, Szudek J, Friedman JM. Use of the National Institutes of Health criteria for diagnosis of neurofibromatosis 1 in children. Pediatrics 2000;105:608–614
3. Sorensen SA, Mulvihill JJ, Nielsen A. Long-term follow-up of von Recklinghausen neurofibromatosis: survival and malignant neoplasms. N Engl J Med 1986;314:1010–1015
4. Zoller M, Rembeck B, Akesson HO, Angervall L. Life expectancy, mortality, and prognostic factors in neurofibromatosis type 1: a twelve-year follow-up of an epidemiological study in Goteborg, Sweden. Acta Derm Venereol 1995;75:136–140
5. North KN, Riccardi V, Samango-Sprouse C, et al. Cognitive function and academic performance in neurofibromatosis 1: consensus statement from the NF1 Cognitive Disorders Task Force. Neurology 1997;48:1121–1127
6. Whitehouse D. Diagnostic value of the café-au-lait spot in children. Arch Dis Child 1966;41:316–319
7. Crowe FW, Schull WJ. Diagnostic importance of café-au-lait spot in neurofibromatosis. Arch Intern Med 1953;91:758–766
8. Friedman JM, Gutmann DH, MacCollin M, Riccardi VM, eds. Neurofibromatosis: Phenotype, Natural History, and Pathogenesis. 3rd ed. Baltimore: Johns Hopkins University Press; 1999
9. Obringer AC, Meadows AT, Zackai EH. The diagnosis of neurofibromatosis 1 in the child under the age of 6 years. Am J Dis Child 1989;143:717–719
10. Huson SM, Harper PS, Compston DA. Von Recklinghausen neurofibromatosis: a clinical and population study in south-east Wales. Brain 1988;111 (pt 6):1355–1381
11. Friedman JM. Neurofibromatosis 1. Gene Reviews [serial online]. September 30, 2002. Available at: *http://www.geneclinics.org.*
12. Evans DG, Baser ME, McGaughran J, Sharif S, Howard E, Moran A. Malignant peripheral nerve sheath tumors in neurofibromatosis 1. J Med Genet 2002;39:311–314
13. Lisch K. Ueber Beteiligung der Augen, insbesondere das Vorkommen von Iris-knotchen bei der Neurofibromatose (Recklinghausen). Z Augenheil 1937;93:137–143
14. Rubenstein AE, Korf BR. Neurofibromatosis: A Handbook for Patients, Families, and Health-Care Professionals. New York: Thieme Medical Publishers; 1990:82

15. Lewis RA, Riccardi VM. Von Reckling-hausen neurofibromatosis: incidence of iris hamartomas. Ophthalmology 1981;88:348–354
16. Huson SM, Jones D, Beck L. Ophthalmologic manifestations of neurofibromatosis. Br J Ophthalmol 1987;71:235–238
17. Zehavi C, Romano A, Goodman RM. Iris (Lisch) nodules in neurofibromatosis. Clin Genet 1986;29:51–55
18. Flueler U, Boltshauser E, Kilchhofer A. Iris hamartomata as diagnostic criterion in neurofibromatosis. Neuropediatrics 1986;17:183–185
19. Listernick R, Charrow J, Greenwald MJ, Esterly NB. Optic gliomas in children with neurofibromatosis type 1. J Pediatr 1989;114:788–792
20. Listernick R, Charrow J, Greenwald M, Mets M. Natural history of optic pathway tumors in children with neurofibromatosis type 1: a longitudinal study. J Pediatr 1994;125:63–66

6

Neurofibromas and Malignant Peripheral Nerve Sheath Tumors (MPNST) in Neurofibromatosis 1

The growth of multiple neurofibromas is not only the hallmark feature of neurofibromatosis 1 (NF1), but also is one of its most complex manifestations. In the century since von Recklinghausen first observed that neurofibromas develop from the myelin sheath of tissue surrounding nerves, researchers have learned much more about how these tumors develop and grow (see Chapter 3). Yet much remains to be learned about these neural tumors, which are so central to the disorder, are responsible for much of its medical complications (morbidity), and cause patients such psychological distress.

This chapter reviews the classification, natural history, and management options for neurofibromas. Although most are benign, some undergo transformation into malignant peripheral nerve sheath tumors (MPNSTs).

◆ Neurofibromas: An Overview

Neurofibromas can develop at any time in life from the tissue surrounding any nerve in the body. Isolated neurofibromas may develop in people without NF1, but multiple neurofibromas develop only in people with the disorder. Some people with NF1 develop only a handful of neurofibromas, whereas others, though they are the minority, develop thousands—and it is unclear why. The rate of growth may also vary. Some neurofibromas cause no physical effects, whereas others may cause discomfort, disfigurement, and functional impairment. The defining feature of NF1, therefore, is one of its most puzzling to clinicians and vexing to patients.

Neurofibroma growth begins in the myelin sheath that surrounds nerves and enables them to send and receive signals more efficiently. As discussed in Chapter 2, electrical impulses are constantly sent back and forth between the brain and spinal cord and the vast peripheral network of nerves that reach every part of the body. This neural communications network enables people to do such things as smell, touch, move, and think. Although it is often compared with the plastic coating in electrical wires, the myelin sheath forms from multiple layers of fatty tissue, which is itself made up of multiple cell types.

The neural tumors in NF1 develop when cells in the protective sheath begin to multiply out of control. This most likely occurs because the tumor suppressing effects of the *NF1* gene are lost (see Chapter 3). Several different neural tumors may develop in NF1. The type of tumor that develops depends on its location in the body and which cells are involved. The most common are discrete and plexiform neurofibromas that develop in the tissue surrounding peripheral nerves (Fig. **6–1**).

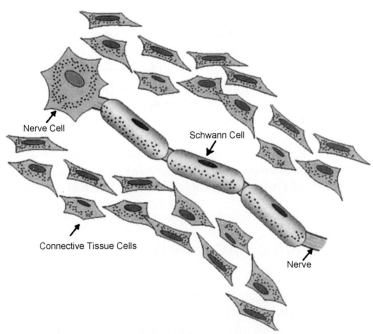

Figure 6–1   Neurofibromas develop from Schwann cells that make up the protective sheath around nerves.

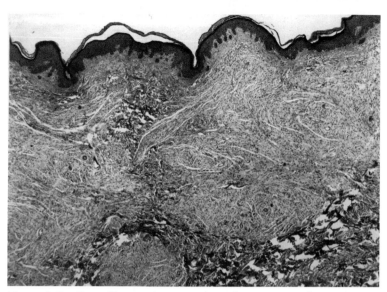

Figure 6–2   Neurofibroma, hematoxylin and eosin–stained section. Low-power view showing nonencapsulated but well-circumscribed spindle-cell tumor in the dermis. (Original magnification, 45×.)

Pathologically, neurofibromas consist of a mixture of many different types of cells, some derived from the nerve sheath itself and others from surrounding tissues and other types of cells (Figs. **6–2** and **6–3**). Spindle-shaped cells proliferate abundantly. These include the Schwann cells that help to form the myelin sheath in the peripheral nervous system, and perineural fibroblasts, which are among the most common types of cells that make up the connective tissue surrounding nerves. The tumors also contain mast cells (inflammatory cells that probably exist in multiple tissue types but seem to be notably drawn to neurofibromas), collagen (the supportive protein component of connective tissue and skin, as well as bone and cartilage), and the extracellular matrix (the substance between cells). As the various cells proliferate, the nerve itself is not usually jeopardized. The axons, fiber-like extensions that enable nerve cells to communicate, pass through the developing neurofibroma tumor mass. This stands in contrast to schwannomas, where the proliferating tumor mass displaces axons and thereby impedes nerve function.

Discrete neurofibromas are encapsulated; they may grow in size and press on other tissue or bone but will not invade them. Plexiform neurofibromas (Fig. **6–4**), on the other hand, are nonencapsulated; they can grow through healthy tissue and interfere with the normal development of bones, which makes management more difficult. Plexiform neurofibromas

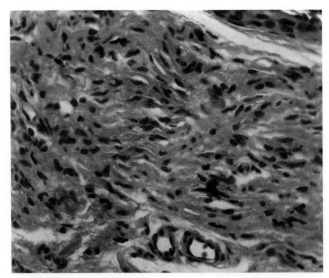

Figure 6–3   Neurofibroma, hematoxylin and eosin–stained section. A high-power view demonstrating the wavy nature of the cells and the curved or S–shaped nuclei. (Original magnification, 500×.)

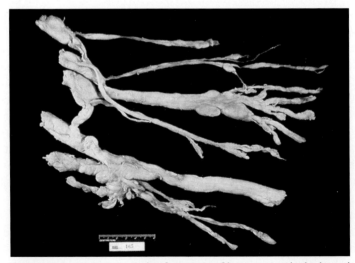

Figure 6–4   A dissected plexiform neurofibroma reveals thickened nerve trunks and multiple extensions of the tumor.

tend to be supported by a network of blood vessels that supply oxygen and nutrients.

A "two-hit" loss of the *NF1* gene (one an inborn mutation and the other an acquired mutation) in Schwann cells probably initiates the formation of a neurofibroma, but loss of function of one copy of the gene in surrounding cells is also necessary before the tumor can grow (see Chapter 3). Hormones may also contribute to the growth of neurofibromas. Discrete dermal neurofibromas usually first develop around the time of puberty. During pregnancy, both discrete and plexiform neurofibromas tend to increase in size, and dermal neurofibromas may increase in number (see Chapter 9). Until recently the hormonal effects on people with NF1 were anecdotal, although quite voluminous. This situation changed when a study reported that three in four neurofibromas contained molecular receptors for the hormone progesterone, a female sex hormone produced by the ovaries during the menstrual cycle and by the placenta during pregnancy.[1] The presence of such receptors indicates that these neurofibromas are sensitive to fluctuations in levels of progesterone and supports the notion that this may be the responsible hormone. It does not, however, completely prove that this hormone (or any hormonal factor) is responsible for neurofibroma growth. Another theory is that additional genetic mutations may contribute to the development and fuel the growth of neurofibromas. The research in this area continues.

From a clinical perspective, there are two basic types of neurofibromas, discrete and plexiform, which each have two subtypes.

Discrete Neurofibromas

A discrete neurofibroma is a benign tumor that arises from a single site on a peripheral nerve and grows into a rounded mass with well-defined borders. These types of neurofibromas generally begin to appear in late childhood or just before puberty and increase in size and number with age. Discrete neurofibromas rarely, if ever, become malignant.

Discrete Cutaneous (or Dermal) Neurofibromas

A discrete dermal neurofibroma is one that develops along a nerve in one of the upper layers of the skin (the dermis or epidermis). As dermal neurofibromas grow, they usually protrude above the surrounding skin surface. At first, they may resemble mosquito bites, but they do not itch or subside. With time they may grow larger. Dermal neurofibromas tend to be soft and fleshy to the touch, and the skin covering them may be flesh-colored, pink, or purple. As dermal neurofibromas grow, they may appear either as a rounded sessile mass rising from a broad base on the skin or as a larger mass attached to the skin with a smaller stalk (pedunculated). They may become lobulated, a single lesion divided into small lobes. Sometimes, dermal neurofibromas that develop in the second or third layer of skin rather than the top one will cause an indentation, and the skin covering them will be violet.

Although dermal neurofibromas can develop anywhere on or in the body, they tend to develop most often on the chest, abdomen, and back, known collectively as the trunk. The most common pattern of growth is slow, with a limited number of neurofibromas appearing just before puberty and then steadily growing in number and size over a period of years. There are exceptions, however. People who have deletion of the whole *NF1* gene (rather than a mutation in part of it) tend to develop a significant number of dermal tumors while they are young. Other people may first develop dermal neurofibromas during their 20s. Sometimes, multiple dermal neurofibromas seem to sprout over a matter of months rather than years. Usually this type of rapid growth subsides. It is also possible that neurofibromas will develop but not progress noticeably during a person's lifetime. Some women experience neurofibroma growth during pregnancy (see Chapter 9). Dermal neurofibroma growth generally continues through middle age and even beyond, but it tends to stabilize when the person becomes elderly.

Depending on their location or number, the major problem that dermal neurofibromas cause is cosmetic, although this term is not meant to trivialize the physical and psychological impact of these lesions. Dermal neurofibromas on the face and neck, and other exposed areas of skin, may be unsightly and cause psychological distress. Dermal neurofibromas are usually not painful, although some people with NF1 experience sharp pain if one is bumped or pressed. Those located on areas rubbed by clothing, such as the collar line or waistline, may cause physical discomfort. Large pedunculated neurofibromas may be accidentally torn off, causing bleeding. Others may be bumped repeatedly, causing pain. That is why some people with NF1 choose to have neurofibromas removed surgically (see below).

Discrete Subcutaneous Neurofibromas

A subcutaneous neurofibroma is a discrete tumor that develops along a nerve contained in deeper body tissue, located under the epidermis. Discrete subcutaneous neurofibromas are usually firm and rubbery to the touch, and may feel like tiny beads beneath the skin. They may be sensitive and painful when pressure is applied. Although subcutaneous neurofibromas are often visible as bumps, the skin can be moved over them to distinguish them from dermal neurofibromas. Such tumors vary in size,

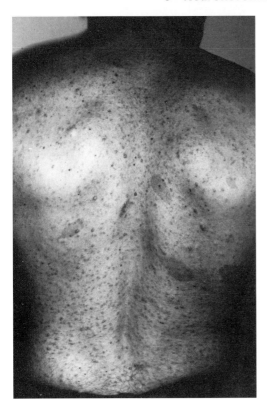

Figure 6–5 Multiple café-au-lait spots and both dermal and subcutaneous neurofibromas on the back of a man with NF1.

ranging from those that are about as large as peas to those that are several centimeters in diameter. Some are so small that they can be "seen" only at an angle, at certain lights, in which the skin takes on a dappled or pebbly appearance (Fig. **6–5**). Other discrete subcutaneous neurofibromas are detected only by palpating the area.

It is also possible for discrete subcutaneous neurofibromas to develop in deeper nerves. With time, these may grow enough to compress a nerve root, causing radicular pain (felt at a site distant from the compromised nerve root) and other symptoms. Unusually challenging, in terms of symptoms and management, are discrete subcutaneous neurofibromas that develop in the tissue surrounding nerve roots within the spinal column (Figs. **6–6** and **6–7**). With time, the neurofibroma can expand on either side of the neural foramen (the opening through which the nerve enters the spinal cord), taking on a dumbbell shape as it grows. Such neurofibroma growth may compress the nerve root, or the spinal cord itself, resulting in radicular symptoms such as weakness in the limbs, loss of sensation, and pain.[2]

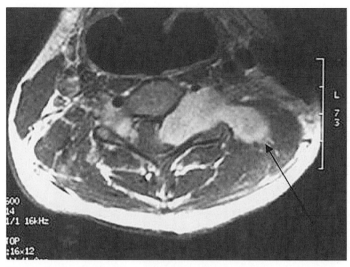

Figure 6–6   Magnetic resonance imaging (MRI) scan showing a spinal neurofibroma.

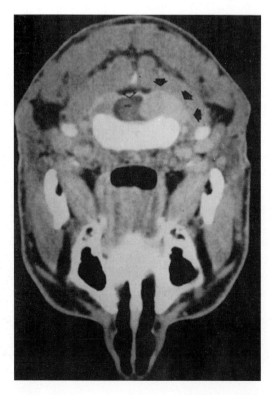

Figure 6–7   This computed tomography (CT) scan demonstrated a spinal root neurofibroma (closed arrows) pressing on the spinal cord (open arrow).

Plexiform Neurofibromas

A plexiform neurofibroma grows along the length of a peripheral nerve sheath, rather than being anchored to a single site within the sheath. Plexiform neurofibromas are usually present at birth (although they may not be noticed), grow during childhood, and then stabilize, although there are some exceptions to this general rule. Though most plexiform neurofibromas are benign, some may develop into MPNSTs.

Diffuse Plexiform Neurofibromas

Most plexiform neurofibromas that develop in people with NF1 are diffuse in nature (Figs. **6–8**, **6–9**, and **6–10**). As the term implies, a diffuse plexiform neurofibroma is one that spreads out from its area of origin. This type of neurofibroma often develops multiple tumor branches that may engulf additional peripheral nerves or extend into adjacent healthy

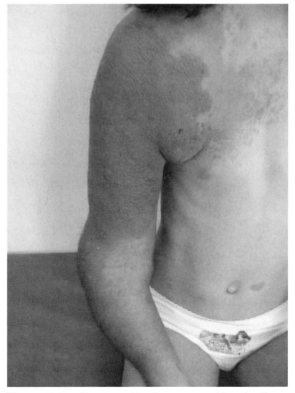

Figure 6–8   Overgrowth of arm caused by plexiform neurofibroma.

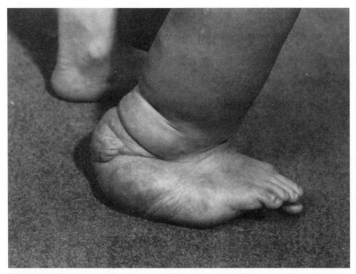

Figure 6–9   A plexiform neurofibroma in the foot or ankle may lead to deformities that severely compromise the function of the extremity.

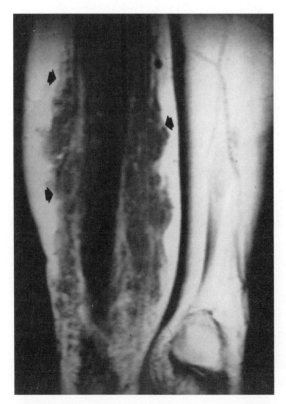

Figure 6–10   MRI of lower legs in a patient with NF1. This longitudinal section shows a leg enlarged by a plexiform neurofibroma (arrows).

tissue. Major nerves as well as minor ones can become involved. In many cases, however, the organization of the nerve itself is preserved so that function is not impaired.[3(p53)]

If diffuse plexiform neurofibromas are located near the surface of the skin, they may feel like a cord-like network when palpated. Sometimes diffuse plexiform neurofibromas are located so deep within the body that they are undetectable by sight or touch, and they may come to attention only when they cause pain or other symptoms. Even diffuse plexiform neurofibromas close to the skin surface may be undetectable if they are small; a discoloration of the skin, similar to a café-au-lait spot, may be the only sign that one exists. In other instances, the skin covering a diffuse plexiform neurofibroma may look markedly different from surrounding skin; it may be darker in color, coarser in texture, and covered with thick, coarse, black hair. Diffuse plexiform neurofibromas may grow so large that they cause hypertrophy, the overgrowth of healthy skin, bone, or other tissue to accommodate the growing tumor mass. In a worst-case situation, this can create physical deformities and sometimes impair vital functions such as breathing.

Diffuse plexiform neurofibromas are probably more common than realized, because many never cause symptoms. One study reported that one in three people with NF1 in Wales had a plexiform neurofibroma that could be detected clinically.[4] Another study, using imaging technology to identify even those plexiform neurofibromas that could not be detected clinically, identified these tumors in the chests of 20% of participants, and in the abdomen or pelvis of 44%.[5]

Although they may not be noticed at first, diffuse plexiform neurofibromas are usually congenital. In a child's first year, they may be visible only as areas with slight skin discolorations, or as subtle overgrowth in soft tissue. For some children, this may be the first clinical sign that they have NF1. Diffuse plexiform neurofibromas tend to grow rapidly during childhood and then stop. The reason for this is not yet known. There are exceptions. Some diffuse plexiform neurofibromas continue to grow into adolescence; others worsen during pregnancy (see Chapter 9).

Some diffuse plexiform neurofibromas can pose management challenges because the tumor tissue is so intertwined with healthy tissue that it is difficult to remove the neurofibroma surgically. Often healthy tissue and even uninvolved nerves must be sacrificed if a diffuse plexiform neurofibroma is to be removed. Even when such removal is possible, it is virtually impossible to remove the entire tumor. Just as a plant that has been pruned will grow additional branches as long as the root remains, so too do some diffuse plexiform neurofibromas grow back following surgery.

The two regions of the body where diffuse plexiform neurofibromas most often develop are the head and neck and the upper chest,[6(p60)] with tumors most often growing along the fifth, ninth, and tenth cranial nerves.[6(p146)] The fifth cranial nerve, the largest of the cranial nerves, is known as the trigeminal nerve and has several divisions or branches. Diffuse plexiform neurofibromas located on the fifth cranial nerve can grow into the eye socket and possibly into the sinus cavity, depending on which branch of the nerve is host to the tumor. If the tumor grows large enough, it may cause the eye to bulge outward and promote overgrowth of the eyelid (Fig. **6–11**). The growing tumor may cause abnormalities in the shape of the greater wing of the sphenoid bone, a wedge-shaped bone at the base of the skull that helps to form the eye socket. Glaucoma, a loss of vision due to increased intraocular pressure, is also a possibility. If the second division of the trigeminal nerve is the site, the diffuse plexiform neurofibroma may extend to the upper jaw and upper gums. When a tumor grows along the third division, the lower jaw, gums, and front two thirds of the tongue may become enlarged.

Diffuse plexiform neurofibromas that occur on the ninth or tenth cranial nerves may alter and impair vital structures in the upper chest area. This region contains the aorta (the largest blood vessel in the body, which delivers oxygenated blood from the heart to additional blood vessels serving the rest of the body). If a tumor originates on the tenth cranial nerve, known as the vagus nerve, it can sometimes extend along the entire length of the nerve, reaching into the central part of the chest and even down into the abdomen.

Other parts of the body may be affected by diffuse plexiform neurofibromas. These tumors may cause bone abnormalities when they develop in limbs.

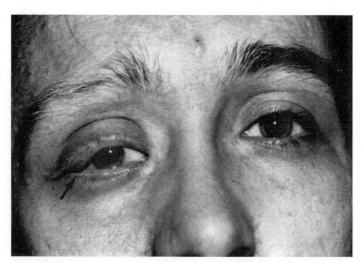

Figure 6–11   A plexiform neurofibroma of the right orbit causes the eyelid to bulge outward.

Nodular Plexiform Neurofibromas

A less common type of plexiform neurofibroma is nodular in nature. A nodular plexiform neurofibroma develops into a focal mass that is similar to a discrete neurofibroma. However, nodular plexiform neurofibromas develop beneath the skin and deep within the body. They cannot be detected by palpation. Multiple nodular plexiform neurofibromas may develop in the same area, dotting a nerve trunk and eventually engulfing it. Such nodular plexiform neurofibromas are usually not detected during childhood; instead, they may come to attention much later, when they begin causing pain, usually when a person with NF1 grows older. In fact, nodular plexiform neurofibromas are more likely than the diffuse type to cause pain.[3(p53)] Some discrete nodular neurofibromas develop from a single nerve root in the spinal column and are known as "dumbbell neurofibromas" because of their distinctive shape as they grow. Because of their location, these may impair movement and present a challenge in management.

◆ Management Options for Neurofibromas

Currently it is not possible to prevent neurofibromas from developing or to retard their growth in any way. Although research is underway to find medical treatments for neurofibromas, it will likely be many years before effective therapies are found. Several surgical options do exist, and some people have experienced good results. There is as yet no consensus, however, about when surgery should be performed or even which option is best. Patients considering surgical removal of neurofibromas should weigh the options carefully to determine which is right for them. It is prudent to consult with a team of physicians, including, surgeons, radiologists, oncologists, and general practitioners, before making any decision.[3(p54)]

Removal of Discrete Neurofibromas

There are several reasons to consider surgical removal of discrete neurofibromas. Dermal neurofibromas may become uncomfortable and painful, depending on their location. Others may become so disfiguring that they bother a patient for cosmetic reasons.

There are several surgical options for removal of discrete neurofibromas; they are explained briefly below. In most cases, surgery can be done on an outpatient basis, using local anesthesia to numb the area. General anesthesia may be necessary if a large number of neurofibromas are to be removed at once. The procedure required depends on the number of discrete neurofibromas to be removed and the difficulty in surgery.

The timing and type of surgery recommended remains controversial. There is no consensus about which is the best approach. Another consideration is that discrete neurofibromas sometimes grow back after surgery in people with a lot of neurofibromas. It is not clear whether the old tumor has grown back or a new one has developed in skin adjacent to the surgical lesion. No long-term studies have been reported to determine whether any one surgical technique is better than the other, or whether any surgical technique attains long-term relief from neurofibromas.

Most health insurers cover the cost of removing discrete neurofibromas, even when removal is done to improve appearance. It is important to work with a physician or surgeon to obtain the proper health insurance approvals and billing codes (see Chapter 14).

Surgical Resection

Plastic surgery involves the removal of a neurofibroma with a scalpel, followed by stitches to close the wound. This generally provides better results than other surgical options, but it may not be practical if a large number of neurofibromas need to be removed. Surgical resection is generally required if the neurofibroma is deeply embedded or larger in size than a pencil eraser.

Carbon Dioxide Laser

This type of laser vaporizes a neurofibroma and may provide an option to someone seeking to remove as many as hundreds of neurofibromas during one medical visit. This option may leave more visible scars and discoloration than surgical resection, however.

Electrical Ablation

Another option for neurofibroma removal is electrical ablation. In this procedure, a surgeon uses a special instrument with a thin point that cauterizes the discrete neurofibroma with an electrical current (Fig. **6–12**). This simultaneously destroys the neurofibroma and seals the wound so that no stitches are necessary (Fig. **6–13**). A scab forms over the area treated and then falls off naturally as the skin heals. Some scarring and discoloration may occur. Hundreds of neurofibromas can be treated at once (Figs. **6–14** and **6–15**).

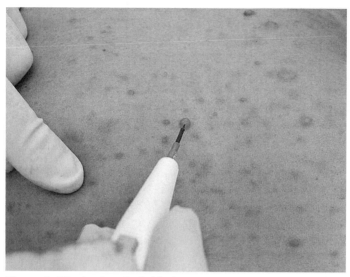

Figure 6–12   In electrical ablation, a surgeon uses a pen-sized instrument to cauterize a dermal neurofibroma. The procedure can be done on an outpatient basis, with local or regional anesthesia. (Courtesy of Hubert Weinberg, M.D., Mt. Sinai School of Medicine, with permission.)

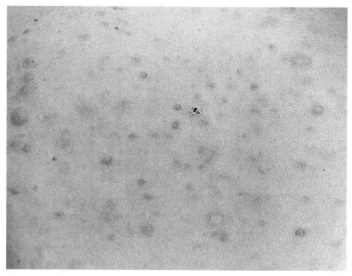

Figure 6–13   A scab will eventually form over the treated area. This falls off naturally as the skin heals. (Courtesy of Hubert Weinberg, M.D., Mt. Sinai School of Medicine, with permission.)

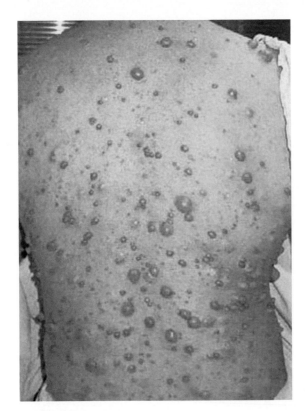

Figure 6–14 A patient with multiple dermal neurofibromas covering the trunk, before electrical ablation is performed. (Courtesy of Hubert Weinberg, M.D., Mt. Sinai School of Medicine, with permission.)

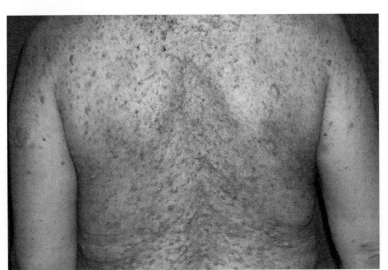

Figure 6–15 Immediately after treatment, the treated neurofibromas have receded and scabs have started to form. Within a week or two, the skin will completely heal. Some areas of treated skin may be slightly darker or lighter than surrounding skin, but this discoloration is usually minor. (Courtesy of Hubert Weinberg, M.D., Mt. Sinai School of Medicine, with permission.)

Removal of Plexiform Neurofibromas

Surgical removal of plexiform neurofibromas is more difficult than removal of discrete neurofibromas because of the nature and structure of the tumors. Plexiform neurofibromas may become intertwined with surrounding healthy tissue, may be full of blood vessels, and may have an irregular, multiprong shape. For this reason, it is usually impossible to completely remove most plexiform neurofibromas. Even partial removal may become difficult if the tumor has entwined itself with vital tissue or nerves. Because the operations are complex, surgery most often is done on an inpatient basis, and it requires general anesthesia.

Although it might be easier to remove a small plexiform neurofibroma, there is no consensus about whether such surgery should be performed. First, there is no guarantee that the tumor will continue to grow; many plexiform neurofibromas stabilize after a period of growth. Second, the smallest plexiform neurofibromas are those in children, but any surgery in children carries its own risks; in any event, there is no guarantee that the tumor will not begin to grow again if any of it remains after surgery.

Even so, there are times when the benefits of surgery for plexiform neurofibromas outweigh the risks. People who are experiencing symptoms such as pain, weakness, or numbness because of a plexiform neurofibroma probably should consider surgery. The decision about whether to operate will depend on how severe the symptoms are and the side effects that may be caused by the operation. If the tumor has grown so that it is intertwined with multiple nerves, surgery itself could cause loss of function or weakness in part of the body. It is also possible that the surgeon can remove part of the plexiform neurofibroma, to alleviate symptoms, while sparing some of the engulfed nerve to preserve function. Nerve grafts may also be attached during surgery to help maintain function if a crucial nerve is sacrificed.

Surgery is also beneficial when the plexiform neurofibroma causes soft tissue overgrowth, resulting in disfigurement and sometimes loss of function in that area. In this case, surgery may improve both appearance and function. A plexiform neurofibroma growing around the eye, for instance, may interfere with vision and the ability to blink the eyelid. A plexiform neurofibroma near the jaw may interfere with speech. A plexiform neurofibroma in the limbs may cause an "elephantine" appearance and interfere with movement. Others are distressing to the patient because they cause disfigurement, which surgery can correct.

Surgery in the head and neck region is especially difficult; the risks of an operation must be weighed against the benefits. Often, several surgical procedures may be required, some to remove the plexiform neurofibroma and others to reconstruct the area. Because plexiform neurofibromas are usually infused with blood vessels, surgery may cause so much bleeding that a blood transfusion is necessary. A common complication of surgery for a plexiform neurofibroma is hematoma, the pooling of blood around the area that has undergone surgery. In that event, a temporary postsurgical drain may be necessary.

The most challenging plexiform neurofibromas to manage surgically are those located in the spine and the brachial plexus, a complicated latticework of nerves located between the neck and shoulder or upper arm. Any operation in these two areas should be carefully considered.

Spinal plexiform neurofibromas occur in many people with NF1, but if they do not cause symptoms, they should be left alone. Those that cause harm are the ones that grow large enough to compress a nerve, causing pain, weakness, and numbness either in the back or elsewhere in the body. Also problematic are those spinal plexiform neurofibromas that grow in a "dumbbell" shape, extending on either side of the neural foramen and thus compressing the spine. These may interfere with bladder and bowel function or impede walking and interfere with mobility. Such tumors usually can be safely and completely removed, but surgery is complicated and requires a long recovery time.

It is more difficult to completely remove a plexiform neurofibroma from within the brachial plexus, the network of nerves that connect the arm and hands to the spinal cord. The nerves in this area are so intertwined that it may be impossible to remove a plexiform neurofibroma without sacrificing function and causing serious disability.

Unfortunately, although the challenges of removing plexiform neurofibromas are well known, the long-term benefits are not. Few studies have looked at long-term outcome, and these report mixed results. One team found that partial removal of plexiform neurofibromas resulted in improvement in one in five people who underwent operations.[7] Another team looked at outcomes at a median of 7 years after surgery, and found that a little more than half (54%) of the plexiform neurofibromas removed did not grow following surgery.[8] More research in this area is needed.

◆ Malignant Peripheral Nerve Sheath Tumors

Sometimes a benign plexiform neurofibroma will become malignant. As discussed in Chapter 3, it is unclear why. Malignant peripheral nerve sheath tumors (MPNST) develop in 5 to 10% of people with NF1.[6(p152),9] MPNSTs sometimes develop in people without NF1, but these tumors are rare in the general population.

Previously, MPNSTs were known as neurofibrosarcomas or malignant schwannomas, terms that reflected the underlying pathology. A rare subtype of MPNST is the triton tumor, which involves malignant transformation of adjacent muscle cells as well as the plexiform neurofibroma.[3(p53)]

The symptoms of MPNSTs vary. If a plexiform neurofibroma starts to grow rapidly, bleeds, or causes pain, the person should contact a physician immediately. When plexiform neurofibromas are located deep within the body, the first symptom of a malignancy is unusual or unexplained pain. Although any plexiform neurofibroma may feel painful for a few hours or even a few days when bumped or injured inadvertently, pain that persists for more than a few days should be investigated. If the malignancy in question develops on a nerve root, the pain may be radicular in nature— felt elsewhere in the body. It is important to be alert to any experience of unexplained pain. Upon palpation, the suspicious plexiform neurofibroma may feel firmer than before, or firmer in some areas than in others. It may grow in size.

Diagnosis can be difficult. Biopsy of suspected tissue, the usual method of confirming a diagnosis in a suspected malignancy, is complicated by the fact that only a small portion of a large plexiform neurofibroma may be malignant. Analysis of excised MPNSTs often reveals cells that have undergone malignant transformation, known as anaplasia, as well as cells that are typical of a neurofibroma. People with NF1 may have multiple plexiform neurofibromas, and any of them may occasionally grow or feel painful.

If an MPNST is suspected, a physician will examine the area, ask about symptoms, and order a magnetic resonance imaging (MRI) scan to better determine if there is an abnormal growth and to guide a biopsy if it is necessary. If the biopsy shows no sign of malignancy, but symptoms continue, a repeat MRI and biopsy may be necessary.

Management Options for Malignant Peripheral Nerve Sheath Tumors

MPNSTs require prompt treatment because these cancers are exceptionally aggressive and tend to metastasize or spread to other parts of the body.[3(p54)] If the MPNST metastasizes, it most often spreads to the lungs. It may also spread to the liver, abdominal cavity, bone, adrenal glands, diaphragm, mediastinum (chest space), brain, ovaries, kidneys, and retroperitoneum (around the membrane that lines the walls of the abdomen and pelvis).

Treatment usually consists of surgical resection, possibly followed by radiation and chemotherapy, especially if the tumor cannot be completely removed. People who are diagnosed early (before the tumor has spread) and are able to have the entire MPNST removed have the best chance of survival. Because MPNSTs present one of the most formidable challenges in management of NF1, diagnosis and treatment should ideally take place at a tertiary hospital (one that engages in patient care, research, and training).

◆ The Personal Perspective

Nancy B.: "As I've grown older, I have developed more skin tumors, neurofibromas, but none that are very large. The larger ones are located where they don't show, so they don't present a cosmetic problem. I'm still a little sensitive about them, though, especially because I have a few small ones on my neck and face that would present a cosmetic problem were they to grow larger. And because NF develops in an unpredictable way, I know they could."

Porter C.: "I did not become disfigured until my early twenties. The tumors started to grow in size and number and continue to do so. When I was about 5, before I had any visible tumors, I was in a play and my character's name was Bumps. If I were superstitious, that caused the NF."

Dolores G.: "Susan had some cranial neurofibromas that had eaten into her skull. She had surgery to remove those and to put some compound on the skull to keep it closed. This required that she have ballooning on the scalp (a medical procedure to expand the skin gradually) so that they could harvest some additional skin. Yet Susan went all through school while handling surgeries. We tried to schedule her surgeries for times like the Christmas holidays so that she wouldn't miss school. She had a large scar on the back of her head, and her hair wouldn't cover all of it. It was difficult for her, but she was bright and perceptive.

"As she grew older, Susan suffered from a lot of internal plexiform neurofibromas, which caused all this pain. She was just filled with internal tumors. A tumor on her bladder was removed, but it returned, so she had extensive bladder surgery."

Tamra M.: "I have one or two neurofibromas on my skin. I have some plexiform tumors on the left facial nerve branch on the left side of my face and down my neck. I've also had them in my spinal cord. That did cause pain about a year ago, in my lower neck, because the tumors were pressing on my nerves within my spinal cord. Then I had surgery on my spinal cord; now it's better.

"The tumor is noticeable in my face. When I was little it wasn't so difficult socially, but then in junior high it was a problem. Some of the kids were rude to me about it, and sometimes I felt self-conscious. We're slowly removing the tumor from my face over time. However, the nerve is now so convoluted through the tumor that if they remove any more I will lose the nerve and not be able to close my eye, or possibly keep the left side of my lips closed. I really don't mind the surgeries. I like the results so far."

References

1. McLaughlin ME, Jacks T. Progesterone receptor expression in neurofibromas. Cancer Res 2003;63:752–755
2. Levy WJ, Latchaw J, Hahn JF, Sawnhy B, Bay J, Dohn DF. Spinal neurofibromas: a report of 66 cases and a comparison with menigiomas. Neurosurgery 1986;18:331–334
3. Gutmann DH, Aylsworth A, Carey JC, et al. The diagnostic evaluation and multidisciplinary management of neurofibromatosis 1 and neurofibromatosis 2. JAMA 1997;278:51–57
4. Huson SM, Harper PS, Compston DA. Von Recklinghausen neurofibromatosis: a clinical and population study in south-east Wales. Brain 1988;111(pt 6):1355–1381
5. Tonsgard JH, Kwak SM, Short MP, Dachman AH. CT imaging in adults with neurofibromatosis 1: frequent asymptomatic plexiform lesions. Neurology 1998;50:1755–1760
6. Friedman JM, Gutmann DH, MacCollin M, Riccardi VM, eds. Neurofibromatosis: Phenotype, Natural History, and Pathogenesis. 3rd ed. Baltimore: Johns Hopkins University Press; 1999
7. Artico M, Cervoni L, Wierzbicki V, D'Andrea V, Nucci F. Benign neural sheath tumours of major nerves: characteristics in 119 surgical cases. Acta Neurochir (Wien) 1997;139:1108–1116
8. Needle MN, Cnaan A, Dattilo J, et al. Prognostic signs in the surgical management of plexiform neurofibroma: the Children's Hospital of Philadelphia experience, 1974–1994. J Pediatr 1997;131:678–682
9. Evans DG, Baser ME, McGaughran J, Sharif S, Howard E, Moran A. Malignant peripheral nerve sheath tumors in neurofibromatosis 1. J Med Genet 2002;39:311–314

7

Other Neural Tumors and Nervous System Abnormalities in Neurofibromatosis 1

As would be expected in a disorder caused by the loss of a tumor suppressor gene, neurofibromatosis 1 (NF1) increases the risk of developing multiple types of tumors in both the central and peripheral nervous systems. Although most NF1-associated tumors are benign neurofibromas (see Chapter 6), the disorder also increases the risk of other types of tumors and certain malignancies. The tumors that arise in the central nervous system (CNS) are potentially more severe in terms of medical impact than are neurofibromas. The CNS tumors most likely to occur in NF1 are optic glioma (a tumor of the optic nerve) and astrocytoma (a type of brain tumor). People with NF1 also develop pheochromocytoma (an adrenal gland tumor), juvenile myelomonocytic leukemia (a blood cancer), and rhabdomyosarcoma (a muscle cell tumor) more frequently than the general population. Because these cancers are all uncommon, the overall risk for someone with NF1 is still low.[1]

In addition, NF1 exerts multiple effects on the developing nervous system, in ways that researchers are only beginning to understand. The most common nervous system abnormalities seen in NF1 are *macrocephaly* (a large head) and headaches. Less frequently, epilepsy and *hydrocephalus* (fluid buildup in the brain) may occur.

This chapter discusses the most common CNS tumors and other malignancies in NF1 and nervous system abnormalities typical of the disorder.

◆ Optic Gliomas

Optic pathway gliomas are tumors that develop from cells known as astrocytes that surround the optic nerve. The tumors are called gliomas because astrocytes are among the most common glial cells in the brain (see Chapter 3). Optic gliomas are common in people with NF1, present in an estimated 15% of people with the disorder, although there is evidence that these tumors occur less frequently in African Americans.[2–4] In most cases, however, the tumors are slow growing, do not cause symptoms, and do not require treatment. Only 5% of children with NF1 develop vision abnormalities related to an optic glioma, for instance.[2] Some children with an optic glioma may experience early puberty, depending on the tumor's location.

Optic pathway gliomas develop in the preschool years, with most presenting between the ages of 4 and 6. For that reason, an annual eye examination by an ophthalmologist is recommended for any child with NF1.[1] Although other types of routine screening, such as magnetic resonance imaging (MRI) scans, are not recommended unless symptoms develop, this remains a controversial issue. Some physicians advocate routine MRI scans to determine whether or not a child with NF1 has developed an optic glioma. The consensus remains, however, that neuroimaging studies may detect asymptomatic tumors, but they do not prevent symptoms from developing, improve treatment, or alter long-term outcomes.[5]

Optic gliomas are low-grade tumors and are usually not aggressive.[6(p235)] They can develop anywhere along the optic nerve, including inside the eye socket (the intraorbital portion of the nerve), inside the skull (intracranial portion), on the optic chiasm (the area in the brain where the optic nerve from each eye crosses before extending further into the brain), or on the optic tracts leading to the visual cortex. Most optic gliomas are found in the intraorbital and intracranial sections of the optic nerve or the optic chiasm.[6(p205)]

Although optic pathway gliomas constitute only 2 to 5% of all childhood brain tumors, children with NF1 have 70% of those that are diagnosed.[6(p203)] It is not clear why optic pathway gliomas occur more often in people with NF1 than in the general population. Analysis of autopsied tissue from people, as well as laboratory studies in mice, indicates that the *NF1* gene mutation, which causes a loss of neurofibromin protein, somehow encourages an increase in the proliferation of astrocytes. The overabundance of these cells contributes to tumor formation (see Chapter 3).

The tumors that progress and cause symptoms quite likely do so because of the influence of hormones and/or of additional genetic mutations.[6(p207)] This theory is bolstered by population-based (epidemiological) studies that have found that in children with NF1 girls are twice as likely to develop an optic glioma as boys.[7,8]

Symptoms and Diagnosis

As many as two thirds[4] of optic gliomas do not cause symptoms. About half[6(p208)] of people who do become symptomatic experience vision abnormalities, but these rarely get worse and can either go without treatment or be managed with eyeglasses. In one in three people with symptomatic tumors, the tumor causes progressive proptosis,[8–10] in which the eye bulges outward. Complete or partial loss of vision may result.

Another potential complication of optic pathway glioma is premature puberty, which results in about one in three children who develop symptoms.[8] Precocious puberty is that which occurs before the age of 7 in girls and 9 in boys.[6(p215)] Early puberty occurs when the optic glioma is located in the optic chiasm and places pressure on the hypothalamus, the area of the brain that controls the secretion of hormones, among other functions. The first sign that a child with NF1 may experience precocious puberty is a sudden growth spurt, so that the child is taller than the normal range for peers (see Chapter 9).

Regular vision examinations help to detect symptoms indicating the presence of an optic glioma. A child with NF1 should be examined by a pediatric ophthalmologist or an ophthalmologist experienced in treating people with NF1. The examination should include an assessment of visual acuity, color vision, and visual fields, as well as examination of the optic nerve and eyeball. Annual visits are recommended for all children with NF1 until 10 years of age,[1] and afterward if an optic glioma or vision irregularity is detected. Asymptomatic older children and adults should also undergo regular eye exams, although how frequently they occur and how extensive they should be may vary. (Ask an NF specialist for personal advice.)

Any of the following symptoms or clinical findings made during an ophthalmological exam may indicate the presence of an optic glioma. However, a normal exam does not rule out the presence of a tumor. Two of three people with an optic glioma have normal vision and other findings on an eye exam.[11(p85)]

Decreased Visual Acuity

Performance on a vision test indicates whether there is vision loss in one or both eyes. This can be a difficult screening test for young children, yet that is the age when the optic glioma is most likely to develop.

Decreased Color Vision

This is another good indication that a tumor may be present on the optic nerve, but it may be difficult to assess in young children.

Afferent Pupillary Defect

When a light is shined suddenly at a normal eye, pupils in both eyes constrict. In an eye with optic nerve damage, however, the pupil may dilate—an indication that the nerve is not functioning properly and the information it conveys to the brain may be garbled.

Visual Field Defects

Defects in the visual field include deterioration of the central or peripheral vision and "blind" spots. Visual field testing is hard to do in children under age 7, those most likely to harbor these defects. Experts recommend that this type of test be reserved for children older than 7 who are known to have lesions in the optic chiasm. In this case, visual defects will be present in both eyes.[6(p205)]

Papilledema

This is a swelling of the optic nerve caused by increased pressure inside the skull.

Optic Nerve Atrophy

When the nerve atrophies, it loses color and mass. Inasmuch as this manifestation occurs after others have become evident, it may not be useful in diagnosis.

Visual Evoked Responses

This test measures electrical activity in the brain's visual cortex to gauge the health of the visual pathways. (The patient watches a monitor with moving patterns while electrodes are attached to the scalp.) Although this test may be useful in evaluating the health of the optic nerve, it does not always reveal the presence of an optic glioma. Many people with such tumors perform normally in the visual evoked response test.

If an eye examination or visual evoked response test reveals telltale vision discrepancies or optic nerve dysfunction, an MRI of the head and eye sockets will reveal whether a tumor is growing along the optic nerve

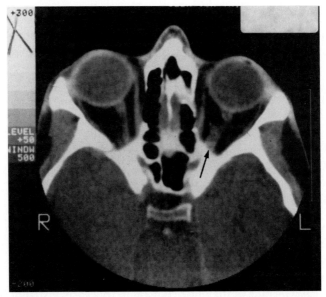

Figure 7–1   Magnetic resonance imaging (MRI) reveals an optic glioma of the left optic nerve (arrow).

(Fig. **7–1**). If the child does have an optic glioma, monitoring should consist of regular follow-up ophthalmological exams, to determine whether symptoms are getting worse, and periodic MRIs as recommended by a physician.

All children with NF1 should have their height and weight measured at least annually and compared with standard growth charts. The first sign that the child will experience premature puberty is accelerated growth in height. This may also be the first sign that the child has an optic glioma, even when vision tests are normal.

Management of Optic Pathway Gliomas

Because most optic gliomas do not progress, become invasive, or cause any symptoms,[3] the best strategy is one of watchful waiting and regular follow-up eye exams.

A small proportion of optic pathway gliomas require treatment because they compromise vision, are disfiguring, or compress adjacent brain structures.[12] Because of the location of these tumors, surgical resection is difficult. The only way to completely remove the tumor is to remove the optic nerve, which would cause blindness in that eye. Sometimes surgery is useful in reducing the size of the tumor (a process known as debulking it).

The mainstay of treatment is chemotherapy, usually with a combination of vincristine and carboplatin, although carboplatin may be used alone.[5,13] If necessary, this initial treatment is followed by radiation, usually when the child is older to minimize long-term side effects. The goal of treatment is to reduce the size of the tumor, retard further tumor growth, and preserve vision. A risk of chemotherapy and radiation is that secondary malignancies may develop, as they sometimes do in other disorders involving loss of a tumor suppressor gene. Radiation may damage blood vessels (see the discussion on moyamoya in the subsection Vasculopathy in Chapter 9), leading to stroke, and may contribute to cognitive difficulties. It may interfere with the brain's ability to produce certain hormones, thereby interfering with the child's growth and development.[11(p86)]

◆ Astrocytomas

People with NF1 may develop other types of astrocytomas, although these other brain tumors occur less frequently than optic gliomas. Some brain tumors are never detected because they cause no symptoms. Others can induce seizures, changes in behavior, loss of sensation, visual disturbances, lethargy, or even coma. Another sign that a brain tumor may be present is recurrent headache, sometimes combined with vomiting. Headaches may occur for many reasons; not every headache is associated with a brain tumor.

If a tumor is suspected because of clinical symptoms, a neurological exam helps to determine what type of functional impairment exists, which provides clues about the tumor's location. Neuroimaging, usually an MRI or computed tomography (CT) scan, can confirm a diagnosis and provide more information about the nature and location of the tumor. Treatment varies depending on the type of tumor, its location, and the overall health of the individual.

◆ Other Malignancies in Neurofibromatosis 1

People with NF1 are at a somewhat increased risk of developing several types of uncommon tumors and malignancies. Because these tumors and cancers occur so infrequently, overall risk of a person with NF1 developing them remains low. The consensus is that routine presymptomatic screening for any of these tumors in people with NF1 is not necessary.[1]

Pheochromocytomas are tumors on the adrenal gland, part of the body's hormone-producing and regulating endocrine system. Although pheochromocytomas are usually not malignant, these tumors can increase the release of two hormones, adrenaline and noradrenaline, into the bloodstream, which increases both heart rate and blood pressure, and may induce other symptoms such as anxiety, sweating, pallor or flushing, excessive perspiration, and headache. The excess hormones may also disturb the body's ability to regulate blood sugar levels. These tumors can be life threatening if the person is injured or undergoes surgery, because pheochromocytomas may release a flood of adrenaline into the bloodstream following either of these events.

Pheochromocytomas are extremely rare in the general population, but occur with greater-than-normal frequency in people with NF1. (Even so, they do not occur often enough to merit routine screening.) It is likely that pheochromocytomas develop when certain cells in the adrenal glands have mutations in both copies of the *NF1* gene, causing complete loss of the protein neurofibromin.[14,15] About 85 to 95% of pheocromocytomas develop in the inner portion of the gland, known as the adrenal medulla,[6(p237)] although they may occur in nerve tissue as well. The average age of diagnosis in someone with NF1 is 38 years.[6(p238)]

If a pheochromocytoma is suspected, a doctor may first order blood and urine tests to measure levels of adrenaline and noradrenaline, and then order an imaging test (MRI or CT) to identify where the abnormality is located. Surgical removal of the tumor is usually the treatment of choice. If the tumor cannot be removed, a physician will prescribe medications to block the effects of the hormones and to control complications such as high blood pressure.

Carcinoid tumors, like pheochromocytomas, secrete excess amounts of hormones. People with NF1 who develop pheochromocytomas are more likely to develop carcinoid tumors—and vice versa—although both types of tumors are uncommon in the NF1 population.[16,17] If one type of tumor is diagnosed, a patient should be asked about symptoms that might indicate the other type has also developed.

Carcinoid tumors are cancers that usually develop in the gastrointestinal tract, although they can occur elsewhere. These tumors secrete a variety of peptides that are involved in digestion. For the most part, these tumors grow slowly and do not cause symptoms for years, if ever. When symptoms do result, it is between the ages of 40 and 60 that they generally become evident.[16,18,19] Black people with NF1 are more prone to have this tumor than are whites.[20] Initial symptoms may include abdominal cramping and changes in bowel movements caused by obstruction of the intestine. If the tumor spreads to the liver, excessive skin flushing and dizziness may develop, probably because of excess release of hormones that dilate blood vessels. Treatment consists of surgical removal of the tumor and treatment with medications to control symptoms such as flushing. If the tumor has metastasized, it is incurable, but the cancer grows so slowly that individuals with this tumor may live for years.

Juvenile myelomonocytic leukemia (JMML), formerly known as juvenile chronic myeloid leukemia, is a rare blood cancer of the hematopoietic cells, which are the precursors of red blood cells. JMML constitutes less than 1% of all childhood leukemias,[21] but as many as 14% of these cancers[22] occur in children with NF1.

It is believed that JMML develops when *NF1* gene function is lost, decreasing levels of neurofibromin, which both activates the Ras pathway (implicated in several cancers) and increases sensitivity to certain growth factors. This chain of events encourages myeloid precursor cells to proliferate out of control.[23,24] As with other types of leukemia, treatment usually consists of chemotherapy. Bone marrow transplantation, though, may be necessary to ensure survival.[25,26]

Rhabdomyosarcomas are aggressive, malignant tumors that develop from myoblast cells, which are precursors of mature muscle cells. These tumors may occur throughout the body, although they most often develop in the head and neck, urinary and reproductive organs, limbs, and trunk. Most rhabdomyosarcomas develop in children and teenagers, with a peak incidence between 1 and 5 years of age.[27]

The tumor may first attract notice because it causes a visible lump. Those that are located deeper in the body cannot be seen, but they may have effects like eye protrusion, if located in the eye socket, or trouble urinating, if located on the bladder.

It is not clear why rhabdomyosarcomas develop, but several lines of evidence suggest that loss or reduction of neurofibromin may prevent myoblasts from differentiating into mature muscle cells. Instead, they proliferate out of control.[28–30] The usual treatment for rhabdomyosarcoma involves surgery, chemotherapy, and radiation. Chemotherapeutic agents include vincristine, cyclophosphamide, dactinomycin, Adriamycin, VP-16, and ifosfamide.[27]

◆ Nervous System Abnormalities

Macrocephaly

For reasons that are unclear, people with NF1 may have a head that is larger in circumference than normal. Studies report that anywhere from 29 to 45% of people with NF1 have large heads, defined as greater than or equal to two standard deviations above the mean for their sex and age.[2,31-33] Skulls are measured at the widest part, known medically as the fronto-occipital circumference. The head is usually enlarged relative to the rest of the body; someone of short stature, for instance, may have a head size in the "normal" range yet out of proportion to his body size. Only rarely is a large skull size related to an underlying disorder such as hydrocephalus (see below). The skull is larger than normal because the brain is also larger than average, although this seems to have no impact on cognition or other manifestations of NF1. The skull remains larger than average throughout the individual's life.

It is not known why the brain and skull grow larger than expected in a significant number of people with NF1. Head size has no correlation with the severity of NF1 symptoms, including cognitive impairment or learning disabilities. Some researchers have reported that children with NF1 have increased white matter (the part of the brain consisting of cells that support the gray matter, which consists of neurons).[34] Autopsies have revealed that people with NF1 have more astrocytes, a type of support cell in the brain, than expected.[35]

Large head circumference should be noted if it occurs and monitored as a child grows older, but it is not cause for worry. The child's skull usually grows at a rate that parallels a normal growth curve. Further evaluation and testing may be necessary if head growth should dramatically accelerate, or if the individual begins to experience headaches, demonstrate neurological abnormalities (such as disturbance of balance), or have papilledema (swelling of the optic nerve because of increased pressure inside the skull). In any of these situations, a thorough neurological exam and possibly an MRI scan can help to determine what may be causing such signs and symptoms.

Headaches

Headaches are common in about one in 10 people with NF1, although these are generally indistinguishable from those experienced in the general population.[32,33] The exceptions to this general rule are headaches associated with some underlying CNS malady such as a brain tumor or a vascular anomaly. Tension headaches that come and go in episodic fashion are the most common type experienced, although people with NF1 may also suffer from migraine headaches. One study found that headaches in individuals with NF1 occurred more frequently between the ages of 7 and 14 and then became less common with age.[36]

If an individual with NF1 experiences multiple headaches, the best strategy for the patient (or parent) is to compile a "headache diary," noting when headaches occur, how long they last, any notable symptoms, and any possible triggers. Note also whether there is a history of headaches among first-degree relatives (parents, siblings, and children). Migraine headaches may cause more than pain. Visual disturbances such as flashing lights, blind spots, or even visual hallucinations are not unusual. Many children with NF1 and migraines also experience stomachaches. If temporary neurological complaints such as limb weakness occur, note this as well.

This information helps the physician to determine whether further testing is necessary. If the headaches are unusually severe or long-lasting, or causing significant problems, the physician may conduct a thorough physical examination, including a neurological and ophthalmological evaluation. Problematic symptoms include partial paralysis, impediment to reading, writing, speaking, or comprehension (collectively known as aphasia), and/or disturbances in perceptions. Depending on the results of the initial examinations, further testing, such as MRI of the brain or a cerebral *angiogram*, may be necessary.

For the most part, however, headaches in people with NF1 are similar to and treated in the same way as headaches in the general population. Tension headaches may respond to over-the-counter pain medication. Management of migraine headaches may involve prevention with medications such as propranolol or amitriptyline and/or treatment of symptoms with medications such as sumatriptan. Reduction of light and stimulus may also help (see the discussion on pain management in the section Management in Chapter 12).

Epilepsy

Epilepsy is reported in anywhere from 3.5 to 7%[2,32,33,37] of individuals with NF1, although in some cases it is related to NF1 and in other cases it is related to some other underlying condition. Epilepsy can cause seizures, convulsions, and sudden alteration of consciousness. It is not clear why epilepsy develops in people with NF1, and for the most part the type of seizures experienced are similar to those seen in the general population. Grand mal seizures, for instance, involve spasms of the trunk and extremities along with a loss of consciousness. Petit mal seizures are more subtle; the person may suddenly stop all activity and stare blankly into space.

If epilepsy is suspected, a physician may order an MRI and an electroencephalogram (EEG), which measures the patterns of electrical activity in the brain. The physician may also order laboratory studies, such as blood and urine analysis, to rule out infections or irregularities with metabolism. In many cases, a first seizure is not treated; instead, the physician waits to see if another occurs. If a diagnosis of epilepsy is made, treatment generally consists of medications that prevent seizures.

Hydrocephalus

The abnormal buildup of fluid in the brain, known medically as *hydrocephalus,* is a possible complication of NF1. If too much fluid accumulates, it can compress areas of the brain, causing neurological difficulties. In people with NF1, hydrocephalus most often develops because of a condition known as aqueductal stenosis, a constriction of the small canal that connects the third and fourth ventricles, fluid-filled cavities within the brain. The constriction prevents cerebrospinal fluid from draining into the spinal cord as it normally would, and hydrocephalus may result. Aqueductal stenosis is revealed in ~1 to 2.5%[2,32,33] of people with NF1, and usually develops between 6 and 35 years of age.[6(p195)]

Although some people with hydrocephalus experience no symptoms, others may contend with headaches, vision changes, speech difficulties, disturbances in gait, and even seizures. Another sign that hydrocephalus may be present is a swelling of the optic nerve caused by intracranial pressure (papilledema), or an abnormal ophthalmological or neurological exam. To determine whether aqueductal stenosis is present, the physician orders an MRI of the brain. Treatment for hydrocephalus involves surgical insertion of a ventricular shunt to drain cerebrospinal fluid.

◆ The Personal Perspective

Diane D.: "When Julie was 2 years old, she was diagnosed with aspiration, a condition where food goes into the lungs rather than to the stomach. No one could figure out why that was happening. We put her on a feeding tube. It still took a while for us to figure out why she was aspirating.

"I kept a daily journal of her symptoms and it went along with her wherever she went—day care, school, and home. We made a simple chart of how much formula she consumed, whether she vomited, what other symptoms there were, and included a place for comments at the bottom. The symptoms varied. She was vomiting constantly. She sometimes vomited seven times a day. She also had problems talking, walking, and eating, with symptoms lasting for up to 2 weeks. When I reviewed the chart with our doctor in Boston, he thought that Julie might have a migraine syndrome. She was almost 4 then, but young enough that she couldn't tell us if she was having headaches. There were all these other neurological signs. So the doctor prescribed propranolol, which helped.

"We kept her on the feeding tube until she was 5, then weaned her off it and she started eating solid food. We went through a period of experimentation with the medications, but it was clear that she had to remain on the propranolol. We increased the dose as she got older. She'll probably be on some type of medication for the migraines for the rest of her life. She's still much more likely to complain about her stomach first rather than a headache. When she first woke up this morning, you could see by the look on her face that she did not feel well. She said, 'Everything is blurry.' Then she sat down to eat and said, 'I can't eat. I feel sick.' People were surprised that Julie developed a migraine syndrome so young. She was just a year old. Usually this type of problem develops in puberty.

"When Julie was 5, the doctors found an optic glioma. So far it has been asymptomatic, but they're monitoring it. She has an MRI and undergoes visual field testing regularly. She also sees an NF specialist in Boston, a neurologist, and an ophthalmologist."

References

1. Gutmann DH, Aylsworth A, Carey JC, et al. The diagnostic evaluation and multidisciplinary management of neurofibromatosis 1 and neurofibromatosis 2. JAMA 1997;278:51–57
2. Huson SM, Harper PS, Compston DA. Von Recklinghausen neurofibromatosis: a clinical and population study in south-east Wales. Brain 1988;111: 1355–1381
3. Hoyt WF, Baghdassarian SA. Optic glioma of childhood: natural history and rationale for conservative management. Br J Ophthalmol 1969;53: 793–798
4. Lewis RA, Gerson LP, Axelson KA, Riccardi VM, Whitford RP. Von Recklinghausen neurofibromatosis II: incidence of optic gliomata. Ophthalmology 1984;91:929–935
5. Listernick R, Louis DN, Packer RJ, Gutmann DH. Optic pathway gliomas in children with neurofibromatosis 1: consensus statement from the NF1 Optic Pathway Glioma Task Force. Ann Neurol 1997;41:143–149
6. Friedman JM, Gutmann DH, MacCollin M, Riccardi VM, eds. Neurofibromatosis: Phenotype, Natural History, and Pathogenesis. 3rd ed. Baltimore: Johns Hopkins University Press; 1999
7. Listernick R, Charrow J, Greenwald MJ, Esterly NB. Optic gliomas in children with neurofibromatosis type 1. J Pediatr 1989;114:788–792
8. Listernick R, Charrow J, Greenwald M, Mets M. Natural history of optic pathway tumors in children with neurofibromatosis type 1: a longitudinal study. J Pediatr 1994;125:63–66
9. Kuenzle C, Weissert M, Roulet E, et al. Follow-up of optic pathway gliomas in children with neurofibromatosis type 1. Neuropediatrics 1994;25: 295–300
10. Lund AM, Skovby F. Optic gliomas in children with neurofibromatosis type 1. Eur J Pediatr 1991;150:835–838
11. Rubenstein AE, Korf BR. Neurofibromatosis: A Handbook for Patients, Families, and Health-Care Professionals. New York: Thieme Medical Publishers; 1990
12. National Institutes of Health. NIH Neurofibromatosis Consensus Conference. Neurofibromatosis Conference Statement. Arch Neurol 1988;45: 575–578
13. Packer RJ, Lange B, Ater J, et al. Carboplatin and vincristine for recurrent and newly diagnosed low-grade gliomas of childhood. J Clin Oncol 1993;11:850–856
14. Gutmann DH, Cole JL, Stone WJ, Ponder BA, Collins FS. Loss of neurofibromin in adrenal gland tumors from patients with neurofibromatosis type 1. Genes Chromosomes Cancer 1994; 10:55–58
15. Jacks T, Shih TS, Schmitt EM, Bronson RT, Bernards A, Weinberg RA. Tumour predisposition in mice heterozygous for a targeted mutation in *NF1*. Nat Genet 1994;7:353–361

16. Griffiths DF, Williams GT, Williams ED. Duodenal carcinoid tumours, phaeochromocytoma and neurofibromatosis: islet cell tumour, phaeochromocytoma and the von Hippel-Lindau complex: two distinctive neuroendocrine syndromes. Q J Med 1987; 64:769–782

17. Wheeler MH, Curley IR, Williams ED. The association of neurofibromatosis, pheochromocytoma, and somatostatin-rich duodenal carcinoid tumor. Surgery 1986;100:1163–1169

18. Yoshida A, Hatanaka S, Ohi Y, Umekita Y, Yoshida H. Von Recklinghausen's disease associated with somatostatin-rich duodenal carcinoma (somatostatinoma), medullary thyroid carcinoma, and diffuse adrenal medullary hyperplasia. Acta Pathol Jpn 1991;41:847–856

19. Ferner RE. Medical complications of neurofibromatosis 1. In: Huson SM, Hughes RAC, eds. The Neurofibromatoses: A Pathogenic and Clinical Overview. London: Chapman & Hall; 1994:316–330. Cited in Friedman JM, Gutmann DH, MacCollin M, Riccardi VM, eds. Neurofibromatosis: Phenotype, Natural History, and Pathogenesis. 3rd ed. Baltimore: Johns Hopkins University Press; 1999:285

20. Burke AP, Sobin LH, Shekitka KM, Federspiel BH, Helwig EB. Somatostatin-producing duodenal carcinoids in patients with von Recklinghausen's neurofibromatosis: a predilection for black patients. Cancer 1990;65: 1591–1595

21. Arico M, Biondi A, Pui CH. Juvenile myelomonocytic leukemia. Blood 1997;90(pt 2):479–488

22. Niemeyer CM, Arico M, Basso G, et al. Chronic myelomonocytic leukemia in childhood: a retrospective analysis of 110 cases. Blood 1997;89:3534–3543

23. Bollag G, Clapp DW, Shih S, et al. Loss of *NF1* results in activation of the ras signaling pathway and leads to aberrant growth in haematopoietic cells. Nat Genet 1996;12:144–148

24. Largaespada DA, Brannan CI, Jenkins NA, Copeland NG. *NF1* deficiency causes ras-mediated granulocyte/macrophage colony stimulating factor hypersensitivity and chronic myeloid leukaemia. Nat Genet 1996;12: 137–143

25. Sanders JE, Buckner CD, Thomas ED, et al. Allogeneic marrow transplantation for children with juvenile chronic myelogenous leukemia. Blood 1988; 71:1144–1146

26. Bunin N, Saunders F, Leahey A, Doyle J, Calderwood S, Freedman MH. Alternative donor bone marrow transplantation for children with juvenile myelomonocytic leukemia. J Pediatr Hematol Oncol 1999;21: 479–485

27. Rhabdomyosarcoma. Association of Cancer Online Resources, Inc. Web site. Available at: http://www. acor.org/diseases/ped-onc/diseases/rhabdo.html.

28. Gutmann DH, Andersen LB, Cole JL, Swaroop M, Collins FS. An alternatively spliced mRNA in the carboxy terminus of the neurofibromatosis type 1 (NF1) gene is expressed in muscle. Hum Mol Genet 1993; 2:989–992

29. Gutmann DH, Cole JL, Collins FS. Modulation of neurofibromatosis type 1 gene expression during in vitro myoblast differentiation. J Neurosci Res 1994;37:398–405

30. Gutmann DH, Geist RT, Rose K, Wright DE. Expression of two new protein isoforms of the neurofibromatosis type 1 gene product, neurofibromin, in muscle tissues. Dev Dyn 1995; 202:302–311

31. Carey JC, Laub JM, Hall BD. Penetrance and variability in neurofibromatosis: a genetic study of 60 families. Birth Defects Orig Artic Ser 1979;15: 271–281

32. North K. Neurofibromatosis type 1: review of the first 200 patients in an Australian clinic. J Child Neurol 1993; 8:395–402

33. Riccardi VM. Neurofibromatosis: Phenotype, Natural History and Pathogenesis. 2nd ed. Baltimore: Johns Hopkins University Press; 1992. Cited in Friedman JM, Gutmann DH, MacCollin M, Riccardi VM, eds. Neurofibromatosis: Phenotype, Natural History, and Pathogenesis. 3rd ed. Baltimore: Johns Hopkins University Press; 1999:191

34. Said SMA, Yeh TL, Greenwood RS, Whitt JK, Tupler LA, Krishnan KR. MRI morphometric analysis and neuropsychological function in patients with neurofibromatosis. Neuroreport 1996;7:1941–1944

35. Nordlund ML, Rizvi TA, Brannan CI, Ratner N. Neurofibromin expression and astrogliosis in neurofibromatosis (type 1) brains. J Neuropathol Exp Neurol 1995;54:588–600

36. Clementi M, Battistella PA, Rizzi L, Boni S, Tenconi R. Headache in patients with neurofibromatosis type 1. Headache 1996;36:10–13

37. Kulkantrakorn K, Geller TJ. Seizures in neurofibromatosis 1. Pediatr Neurol 1998;19:347–350

8

Cognitive Function and Learning Disabilities in Neurofibromatosis 1

Neurofibromatosis 1 (NF1) impacts brain development in ways that researchers are still trying to understand. About half of all people with NF1 manifest some type of cognitive impairment, also known as a learning disability. This does not mean that people with NF1 are not intelligent. In fact, both the medical and legal definitions of learning disabilities require that someone be of average or above-average intelligence. Individuals diagnosed with NF1 are significantly more at risk than the general population for developing a learning disability or behavioral disorder such as attention deficit disorder (ADD), and slightly more at risk for mental retardation. In fact, cognitive impairment is the most frequent manifestation of NF1 during childhood and often the biggest concern for parents. Fortunately, science has punctured many of the longstanding myths about the cognitive abilities of children with NF1, and there are resources to assist people with the disorder in striving to reach their potentials.

This chapter reviews the cognitive profile of people with NF1, shows how cognitive impairments may be revealed in learning or behavior, and provides practical advice on how to obtain help for someone who has learning disability.

◆ The Neurofibromatosis 1 Cognitive Profile

Scientific understanding about the frequency and nature of cognitive disability in people with NF1 has changed markedly during the 1990s. Although children with NF1 have, on average, an IQ that is lower than the average for the general population, some children with NF1 are of average or above-average intelligence.[1(p1122)] Children with NF1 have a mean IQ (the arithmetic average) between 89 and 94 according to various studies,[2-4] compared with the general population range of 90 to 110. Researchers have not found any correlation between IQ and other NF1 manifestations, gender, or socioeconomic status. One team did find that IQ for children with NF1 increased with age, rising from an average of 90 in children between the ages of 6 and 17, to 99.3 for those 17 years or older.[5] Other studies, though, suggest that there is no improvement in IQ[3] or overall cognition[6] with age. This remains an issue requiring further investigation.

Studies conducted decades ago overestimated the incidence of mental retardation in persons with NF1. Usually the researchers relied on data collected from institutionalized patients and therefore did not include individuals with NF1 living in the community who had milder manifestations of the disorder.[1(p1121)]

About 3% of people in the general population are born with global developmental delay (mental retardation),[1(p1121)] defined as an IQ that is less than 70. Studies done in the past two decades have reported that anywhere from 3% (based on a population-based study)[7] to 5 to 8% (based on IQ measurements made in the clinical setting)[2,3,8] of children with NF1 have global developmental delay. Thus, children with NF1 are *somewhat* more likely to be mentally retarded than the general population, but the risk is not as great as once feared.

Many children with NF1 have some type of cognitive impairment, however. A cognitive impairment is a defect in any brain function, such as the ability to pay attention or process sounds and other aspects of language, which in turn alters the capacity to think and learn. For this reason, cognitive impairment often manifests as a specific learning disability. This general term refers to any one of several hindrances to learning that are not caused by some underlying loss of sight, hearing, motor deficit, mental retardation, or the like. For instance, a child may have normal eyesight and muscle strength, yet have an impairment in the brain's ability to integrate visual input with motor skills. This can result in difficulty with handwriting or coordination. Learning disabilities often impede competence in listening, thinking, speaking, reading, writing, spelling, or doing mathematics. A cognitive impairment may also manifest as a behavioral disorder such as ADD. Although often associated with children, both learning disabilities and behavioral disorders can persist into adulthood.

◆ Learning Disabilities: Myths and Realities

Everyone has a unique learning style. Some people are better at math and science, others at languages. Such variations are completely normal and reflect subtle underlying differences in how individual brains function. These differences are considered "dysfunctions," and therefore cause for concern, when they are pronounced enough to delay brain maturation or age-appropriate skill development. Should this occur, the underlying brain dysfunction has caused a learning disability.

Years ago, many children with learning disabilities were dismissed as "stupid" or criticized for not trying hard enough. Others were seen as obstinate and as behavior problems. Some were even characterized as mentally retarded. As research into the brain and different learning styles progressed, however, physicians and educators came to realize that children with learning disabilities are of average or above-average intelligence, but they require some type of assistance or accommodation to learn. These accommodations function somewhat like eyeglasses for the brain: the goal is to adjust for an inborn difference that interferes with learning. Although there are multiple types of learning disabilities, they generally fall into one of four categories:

- Difficulties with receiving sensory information (visual difficulties, hearing problems)
- Variables in processing the information
- Defects in the brain process of storing and retrieving memories so that information can be "remembered"
- Inability to clearly express what is known (speech impediments, motor coordination impairments)

A child with a learning disability may see letters and numbers on a page as upside down or reversed; an "m" might be seen as a "w," or an "E" as the number "3." Or the child may be unable to organize schoolwork or follow directions. If a motor impairment is involved, handwriting may be illegible.

◆ An Overview of Learning Disabilities in Neurofibromatosis 1

Estimates of the prevalence of learning disabilities in the general population vary. The Centers for Disease Control estimates that 8% of children ages 6 to 11 have a learning disability, and that half of them have ADD as well.[9] Other sources estimate that as many as 20% of people in the United States have a learning disability.[10]

Whatever figure is used, people with NF1 clearly have a higher incidence of learning disabilities than the general population. Various studies have reported that anywhere from 30 to 65% of children with NF1 have learning disabilities.[1(p1122)] The variation probably reflects different definitions of what constitutes a specific learning disability, as well as different methods of collecting data. As is typical of the general population, boys with NF1 are more likely than girls with the disorder to have a learning disability. Some of the latest research disputes this discrepancy between boys and girls and attributes it to cultural biases and/or testing methodologies. Children who come from lower socioeconomic groups are also more at risk. The overall consensus is that about half of all children with NF1 develop some type of learning disability.[11]

Pathology of Learning Disabilities

Because learning disabilities occur so frequently in children with NF1, it is likely that the *NF1* gene mutation may be to blame, although it is not clear how. Neurofibromin exerts its effects in the body by activating certain signaling pathways that direct cell growth and development. Two pathways under investigation for causing learning disabilities are the Ras pathway and the cyclic adenosine 3',5'-monophosphate–protein kinase A (cAMP-PKA) pathway, which both relate to functioning of neurons in the brain, but in different ways.

Researchers studying mice have found, for instance, that excessive Ras activity interferes with the process of learning and memory formation. They theorize that in people with NF1 a similar defect may underlie at least some of the cognitive deficits.[12] A competing theory, based on experiments in fruit flies, is that the cAMP-PKA pathway is responsible for learning deficits. Fruit flies genetically engineered to have one malfunctioning *NF1* gene are worse at learning to escape from a container than normal flies. They also experience defects in potassium channel function, which determines how well signals are sent between neurons.[13–16]

Analysis of neurofibromin's functioning in human brain tissue has provided still other clues. One theory is that neurofibromin helps neurons to send signals to one another, and that a deficiency in the protein may disrupt communication in the brain. Other evidence suggests that neurofibromin contributes to healthy development of particular parts of the brain during the prenatal period.[17] Another developmental theory focuses not on neurons, but on glial cells, the myriad support cells in the brain. Glial cells help form the protective myelin sheath around nerves and mop up excess neurotransmitters—which helps neurons to communicate better. Some scientists propose that loss of neurofibromin causes abnormal growth and development of glial cells.[1(p1124)] The research continues; for now the theories remain speculative.

The Debate About Unidentified Bright Objects

Magnetic resonance imaging (MRI) technology uses radio waves and a strong magnet to produce images of soft structures inside the body, including the brain. Because different tissues emit radio signals of varying intensity, the image that emerges is full of dark and light contrasts, similar to a photograph, that enable brain structures or abnormalities to be seen by someone who is trained to read the scans.

Sixty to 70% of children with NF1 have unidentified bright objects (UBOs) visible on MRI brain scans (Fig. **8–1**). Technically, UBOs are areas of

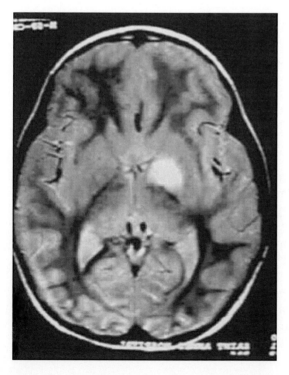

Figure 8–1 An example of an unidentified bright object, or enhanced T2 signal, on magnetic resonance imaging.

increased signal intensity on T2-weighted MRI images. They have no mass and are not known to impede function. Although UBOs can appear anywhere, they most often are located in the basal ganglia, optic tracts, brainstem, and cerebellum. UBOs tend to disappear when people with NF1 reach their 20s or 30s.[1(p1123)]

It is not clear what causes UBOs, although clues are offered by two small studies involving analysis of three brains each. In one, researchers found that brain tissue taken from people with NF1 contained levels of a protein known as gliofibrillary acidic protein (GFAP) that were four to 18 times higher than normal.[18] Such dramatically increased levels of GFAP indicate that a process known as reactive astrocytic gliosis—a change in the number, size, and characteristics of the glial cells that normally support neurons—has taken place. Reactive astrocytic gliosis occurs whenever there is an injury, infection, or abnormality in neurons, and it has been observed in neurodegenerative conditions such as Alzheimer's disease, Parkinson's disease, and Down syndrome.

The other study compared findings on previous MRI studies with analysis of brain tissue on autopsy. The researchers reported that UBOs were found in areas of the brain where there were abnormalities in glial cell proliferation, and the protective myelin sheath had small openings or *vacuoles*, possibly due to swelling and water retention in the myelin (intramyelinic edema). The scientists theorize that UBOs, therefore, may be caused by excess water content or defects in myelin.[19] The research continues.

It is also not yet clear what UBOs signify. They are not correlated with overall severity of NF1, specific neurological deficits, or macrocephaly.[2,20] Some evidence does suggest that UBOs may have some correlation with cognitive impairment, although this is an area that remains controversial and there is no consensus about specifics.

The first studies to examine the question found no relationship between UBOs and cognitive defects. Some critics questioned the scientific methods used, however. Two early studies, for instance, did not consistently measure cognitive function, or even clearly define what skills were being assessed. More recent studies compared detailed medical records, including measures such as IQ scores, with MRI scans. One study found that children with NF1 and UBOs had significantly lower IQ scores than peers with NF1 but without UBOs.[2] Another study, comparing children with NF1 to unaffected siblings, found that the number and size of UBOs was highly correlated with lower IQ scores. The size of UBOs seen in the basal ganglia also had some association with the degree of visuospatial abnormalities a child experienced.[4,21,22] Several other studies, however, have contradicted these results and found no association between UBOs and lower IQ.[23,24] To further muddy the waters, a recent study found that the best predictor of cognitive dysfunction in adulthood was the presence of UBOs in childhood, but that cognition does not improve as the lesions decrease or disappear with age.[6] The debate on this issue continues.

◆ Types of Learning Disabilities in Neurofibromatosis 1

Generally speaking, there is no "learning disability profile" for a child with NF1, although children with the disorder do tend to be weak in mentally processing spoken and written words, numbers, and achieving visuomotor coordination. Contrary to what was suggested by earlier studies, language-based learning difficulties, such as reading and spelling, are as common as nonverbal learning deficits, such as impulsive behavior and poor organizational skills.[2,4,25,26] Children with NF1 tend to perform especially poorly on tests of visuospatial coordination, such as the judgment of line orientation, but many other types of learning disabilities are also common.[11] Usually these differences are discovered when the child enrolls in school and has difficulty completing tasks or understanding what is expected. The first sign of a learning disability in preschool children may be clumsiness (if there is a motor difficulty) or speech delays or difficulty (if related to verbal ability).[27]

None of these learning obstacles reflect poorly on the child's innate intelligence. As the NF1 Cognitive Disorders Task Force stated in its consensus statement, "Simply put, a [specific learning disability] represents a major discrepancy between ability (intellect or aptitude) and achievement (performance)."[1(p1121)] Left untreated, learning disabilities can have lifelong impact on education, career, and overall achievement. Fortunately, remedial interventions are effective and often available free of charge through the school system.

The most common types of learning disabilities seen in NF1 are briefly described below.

Language-Based Learning Problems

Language-based learning disabilities interfere with a person's ability to hear, see, process, or speak words. This type of disability can limit the ability to listen, speak, read, and write. Specific examples include a tendency to reverse or rotate words and letters (mistaking "dog" for "god"), difficulty distinguishing one word or math problem from others on the page, or incorrect word articulation.

Because language is essential to communication, language-based learning disorders can have lifetime impact. They increase a person's risk of doing poorly in school, at work, and in social situations. Typically people with NF1 who have a language-based learning disability may display the following characteristics:

Poor Listening Skills

The individual is easily distracted, has trouble listening to someone for an extended period, or may need longer than other people to "process" what is being said.

Faulty Word Memory

The individual cannot remember grammatical rules or sequences of words.

Limited Reading and Word Comprehension Skills

The individual does not understand what he reads, has a limited vocabulary, and does not understand that the same word sometimes has different meanings. This limits the ability to grasp concepts such as metaphors, irony, and ambiguities.

Difficulty in Verbal Reasoning

The individual finds it hard to understand mathematical word problems or to solve problems verbally.

Impaired Verbal Social Skills

The individual sometimes uses inappropriate language when interacting with others and may misinterpret what another person is saying.

Trouble Distinguishing Sounds

The individual is unable to distinguish between similar-sounding sounds and words, and as a result may misunderstand what is being asked.

Disorganized Communication Skills

The individual may say something that makes no sense or tell a story in which chronological events are out of order.

Nonverbal Learning Disabilities

Nonverbal learning disabilities are those that involve any brain functions *other* than those involved in processing language. This category also encompasses the brain's ability to process and integrate multiple streams of information at once. Examples of nonverbal learning disabilities include visuospatial coordination, motor coordination, perception, and attention.

Visuospatial Coordination

The individual may have difficulty with directions or with orienting himself to surroundings. The person may also have trouble reading and drawing maps, charts and graphs, and diagrams.

Visuomotor Coordination

The individual may be clumsy and tend to bump into things or knock items over when reaching for them. The person also has difficulty with some sports that require hand–eye coordination such as baseball or basketball.

Mixed Learning Disabilities

Certain skills require both verbal and nonverbal abilities. Two notable examples are mathematics and written language. Children with written language disabilities may have poor handwriting, trouble with spelling and grammar, and be unable to compute mathematical equations or solve word problems.

◆ Management of Learning Disabilities in Neurofibromatosis 1

Many middle-aged and older adults with NF1 have faced a lifelong struggle with learning disabilities because they grew up and went to school before such disabilities were recognized as clinical entities, and before public schools were required to provide remedial help. Fortunately, both science and public policy have evolved so that children with learning disabilities can receive the help they need to achieve more of their potential.

Given the high risk that a child with NF1 will develop a learning disability, parents and physicians alike should be alert for signs that a child is not keeping up with normal developmental milestones (the first word, the first step, etc.) and seek appropriate screening. It is important to remember that learning obstacles may develop at any time during the preschool or school-age period, because the nature of learning disabilities varies greatly in type and severity. Differences in ability become evident in some children early in life, but in others they become apparent only as school or intellectual demands increase with age.

If a learning disability is suspected, the child should be evaluated as early as possible by appropriate professionals. Remedial services should be obtained to maximize the child's ability to learn and minimize the chances of falling behind in school.[11] Learning disabilities are usually diagnosed in school-aged children. If a parent suspects a child with NF1 has a learning disability, the first step is to talk with the teacher or school principal to learn what procedures the school has in place. Generally speaking, school officials will conduct standardized tests that measure how the child's skills and abilities compare with what is considered normal. Parents must first be apprised of such testing and what it will involve. They then provide written permission before it can proceed.

Because children with NF1 may have neurological abnormalities, it is important that the child undergo (if he hasn't already) a detailed neurological examination, ophthalmological exam, and hearing test to rule out these sorts of abnormalities. By the time they reach school, children with NF1 should have undergone all of these tests (see Chapter 5). MRI scans are not recommended as part of a routine diagnostic workup for learning disabilities. These scans may be appropriate when the child has a neurological deficit that suggests the presence of a tumor, intracranial pressure, or some other lesion.

After administering the standardized tests, a team of school professionals meets with parents (with the child present, if appropriate) to discuss the results. Generally this team consists of the child's regular teachers, a special education teacher if applicable, school administrators, and other professionals, such as a speech therapist or school psychologist, as required. This same team also determines the child's eligibility for special education services.

A child is eligible for special education services under the provisions of the Individuals with Disabilities Education Act (IDEA, Public Law 101–476). This 1990 law supplanted an earlier law, the Education for All Handicapped Children Act (Public Law 94–142). IDEA covers private as well as public schools and provides criteria for 13 categories of disabilities that are eligible for services. Children with NF1 generally qualify for services under two categories: "specific learning disability" or "other health impairment."

It is important to note that not all children who have a learning difficulty meet the criteria for a "specific learning disability" under IDEA. Nonverbal learning disabilities, for instance, are not eligible for special education services under this category. Children with NF1 who have nonverbal learning disabilities, or have other learning challenges not classified as specific learning disabilities by IDEA, however, may still be able to receive services because NF1 falls under the classification of "other health impairment."

If it is determined that the child is not eligible for services under IDEA, parents must be informed in writing by the school and provided with information about whom to contact to appeal the decision. If this information is not provided, parents should ask for it. Many school districts apply a narrow interpretation of eligibility to avoid the expense associated with providing special education services. Therefore, parents should expect to fight hard for the services their child needs. Many have to be persistent and act as advocates through a lengthy appeals process.

If a child is eligible for services, IDEA stipulates that an individualized education plan (IEP) be developed. An IEP is a written agreement between parents and school officials about what services the child needs. It includes an assessment of the child's abilities, establishes short-term and annual goals for the child, and details the type of services the child will receive to help attain those objectives. The IEP is reviewed at least once a year to review progress and make further adjustments. (Parents can appeal school officials' recommendations and findings. Check with the school district for details.)

Services and accommodations vary, depending on the child's needs. Children with weak visuomotor coordination, for instance, may benefit from treatment by an occupational therapist. Children who are not proficient in organizing information or work may need help to break a task into clearly defined steps. Reading skills can sometimes be improved by having the child read out loud, because the part of the brain that processes spoken words is different from the one that interprets written words. Sometimes the child's teacher can adjust instruction style to meet the child's needs; at other times a special education teacher or teacher's aide may be required to provide the assistance.

Although school systems are usually the primary source for services, they are not the only resources available. Several national and state organizations exist, some with a broad mission and others focused on selected learning disabilities such as dyslexia.

◆ **Behavioral Problems**

Children with NF1 tend to exhibit troubling behavioral patterns such as acting out at others, inflexibility when confronted with change, or a tendency to become distracted and lose focus. Some of these behaviors may result from frustration at not being able to keep up with peers, especially if the child has a learning disability and is not able to interpret and process information as rapidly or efficiently as other children do. At other times, children with NF1 may act out because of a behavioral disorder—with or without a coexisting learning disability. The most common behavioral disorder in children with NF1 is ADD.

According to the *Diagnostic and Statistical Manual of Mental Disorders*, 4th edition (DSM-IV), the standard reference used to diagnose psychiatric and behavioral disorders, a person has ADD if six or more symptoms of inattention persist for at least 6 months. Typical symptoms include failure to pay attention, careless mistakes, problems in organizing work, tendency to become distracted, and difficulty listening even when addressed directly.[28]

If a child is diagnosed with ADD, treatment usually consists of a combination of behavioral interventions and medications. Stimulants are most often prescribed because they activate parts of the brain that are inactive in ADD and help the child to focus. As is the case with learning disabilities, many resources exist to help children with ADD. Parents should consult first with their child's pediatrician and teacher, and then contact both national and local organizations for more information. Such resources can be located with the help of a local librarian or by conducting an Internet search.

◆ When Problems Persist into Adulthood

Learning disabilities are lifelong disabilities. Some people find ways to compensate for them, but adults with NF1 may continue to endure the consequences of learning disability. In some cases, their cognitive differences were not diagnosed and treated appropriately. Many middle-aged and elderly people with NF1 attended school before such cognitive difficulties were understood, treatment was available, or their treatment mandated by law. Insufficient reading and writing skills bar many adults with learning disability from work they would otherwise be capable of and interested in doing. An adult with learning disability may struggle to keep pace with fellow employees or acquire new skills in the workplace.

ADD often persists into adulthood, although this has only recently been recognized. Adults with ADD may make careless mistakes at work, are perceived to be disorganized, or interrupt others in meetings.

Learning disabilities and ADD often manifest themselves more subtly in adults than in children. Because of the frustration they experience each day, adults with learning disabilities and ADD may be discontented with personal relationships and may engage in alcohol or substance abuse.

Fortunately, resources and help have become available, now that adult learning and behavioral maladies are recognized as real—and avoidable. The Americans with Disabilities Act, for instance, mandates that employers make reasonable accommodations for employees with these disorders. For more information, contact a primary care physician or an employee assistance program, which may be available in many large companies.

◆ The Personal Perspective

Diane D.: "Julie was diagnosed with learning disabilities early on, and more recently with attention deficit hyperactivity disorder (ADHD). She started off in early intervention when she was a year old and then transitioned to the school system. The school has been cooperative. But now with ADHD, things have become more challenging. For the past 4 months, Julie's been struggling to find medications she can tolerate. And we're working with the school to see if we can make some adjustments.

"We are working with a person outside the school system, a psychologist who specializes in treating ADHD combined with learning disabilities. She's a tremendous advocate and in close contact with our pediatrician. We've come up with a wonderful team. We are in discussions with the school about changing Julie's learning environment, though. We'll see how that goes."

Dolores G.: "Susan's coordination was a bit questionable. She was klutzy, but so am I, so we didn't think anything about that. She went to preschool and nursery school, and she appeared to be learning well. Her dexterity was bad, but that was attributed to the klutziness. At the time they didn't know much about learning disabilities.

"As she got into middle school, her handwriting was atrocious. Her math and spelling abilities were very bad, but she was a determined child and she made it through. In the fifth grade, she really needed more attention, so we put her into a private school and she went there for 2 years. But the private school wouldn't accept her to its junior high because academically she wasn't adequate. She went back to the public school. But they wouldn't let her enter into her class in junior high. They kept her back a year, which was a real psychological blow to her.

"In high school, Susan did well. She got private tutoring for math and had that for many, many years. She graduated from high school, even though she had a lot of surgeries and was out of school a fair amount of time. Susan had a guidance counselor at school. When she was a junior in high school, he told her, 'Susan, I would suggest that you not try to go to college. You'll be lucky if you make it through trade school.' And she looked at him, and said a few choice words, and then said, 'I am not going to do what you say. You cannot convince me that I'm not going to make it. I'm going to go ahead and take my regular courses.'

"I think it's important for other families to know this in case they encounter something similar. Susan attended Wright State University in Ohio. It's a state school that specializes in young people who are challenged. Some have learning disabilities and others have physical disabilities. Susan did well. She went through the whole program and graduated. It took her 5 years, but not because of academic reasons. She had to take time out from class to undergo surgeries."

Tamra M.: "I've had some small motor skill difficulties. I have trouble writing, so I type or have kids take notes for me in class. I do fairly well in school.

"Last year, I missed practically all of one semester at school because of surgery. I had to wear a head "halo" brace for 8 weeks. I did a home tutoring program and still got credit for all but one of my classes.

"I want to go to college. That's a definite. I want to write. I like to write. I write poetry and fantasy, like *Lord of the Rings*. I am taking a creative writing class now, and am enjoying it. It's fun. I've had two poems published. One was in an NF newsletter and the other was in my school's magazine."

References

1. North KN, Riccardi V, Samango-Sprouse C, et al. Cognitive function and academic performance in neurofibromatosis 1: consensus statement from the NF1 Cognitive Disorders Task Force. Neurology 1997;48: 1121–1127
2. North K, Joy P, Yuille D, et al. Specific learning disability in children with neurofibromatosis type 1: significance of MRI abnormalities. Neurology 1994;44:878–883
3. Ferner RE, Hughes RA, Weinman J. Intellectual impairment in neurofibromatosis 1. J Neurol Sci 1996;138: 125–133
4. Hofman KJ, Harris EL, Bryan RN, Denckla MB. Neurofibromatosis type 1: the cognitive phenotype. J Pediatr 1994;124:S1–S8
5. Riccardi VM. Type 1 neurofibromatosis and the pediatric patient. Curr Probl Pediatr 1992;22:66–106
6. Hyman SL, Gill DS, Shores EA, et al. Natural history of cognitive deficits and their relationship to MRI T2-hyperintensities in NF1. Neurology 2003;60:1139–1145
7. Huson SM, Harper PS, Compston DA. Von Recklinghausen neurofibromatosis: a clinical and population study in south-east Wales. Brain 1988;111 (pt 6):1355–1381
8. Moore BD, Ater JL, Needle MN, Slopis J, Copeland DR. Neuropsychological profile of children with neurofibromatosis, brain tumor, or both. J Child Neurol 1994;9:368–377
9. Department of Health and Human Services, Centers for Disease Control and Prevention, National Center for Health Statistics. Attention deficit disorder and learning disability: United States, 1997–1998 data from the National Health Interview Survey May 2002

10. Learning disabilities. Fact sheet 7, January 2003. National Information Center for Children and Youth with Disabilities Web site. Available at: http://www.nichcy.org/pubs/factshe/fs7txt.htm.

11. Gutmann DH, Aylsworth A, Carey JC, et al. The diagnostic evaluation and multidisciplinary management of neurofibromatosis 1 and neurofibromatosis 2. JAMA 1997;278:51–57

12. Costa RM, Federov NB, Kogan JH, et al. Mechanism for the learning deficits in a mouse model of neurofibromatosis type 1. Nature 2002;415:526–530

13. Guo HF, The I, Hannan F, Bernards A, Zhong Y. Requirement of Drosophila NF1 for activation of adenylyl cyclase by PACAP38-like neuropeptides. Science 1997;276:795–798

14. Guo HF, Tong J, Hannan F, Luo L, Zhong Y. A neurofibromatosis-1-regulated pathway is required for learning in Drosophila. Nature 2000;403:895–898

15. The I, Hannigan GE, Cowley GS, et al. Rescue of a Drosophila NF1 mutant phenotype by protein kinase A. Science 1997;276:791–794

16. Cichowski K, Jacks T. NF1 tumor suppressor gene function: narrowing the GAP. Cell 2001;104:593–604

17. Gutmann DH. Recent insights into neurofibromatosis type 1: clear genetic progress. Arch Neurol 1998;55:779

18. Nordlund ML, Rizvi TA, Brannan CI, Ratner N. Neurofibromin expression and astrogliosis in neurofibromatosis (type 1) brains. J Neuropathol Exp Neurol 1995;54:588–600

19. DiPaolo DP, Zimmerman RA, Rorke LB, Zackai EH, Bilaniuk LT, Yachnis AT. Neurofibromatosis type 1: pathologic substrate of high-signal intensity foci in the brain. Radiology 1995;195:721–724

20. Duffner PK, Cohen ME, Seidel FG, Shucard DW. The significance of MRI abnormalities in children with neurofibromatosis. Neurology 1989;39:373–378

21. Denckla MD, Hofman K, Mazzocco MM, et al. Relationship between T2-weighted hyperintensities (unidentified bright objects) and lower IQs in children with neurofibromatosis 1. Am J Med Genet 1996;67:98–102

22. Mott S, Kkryja PB, Baumgardner T, Abramson A, Reiss A, Denckla M. Neurofibromatosis type 1 (NF1): association between volumes of T2-weighted high intensity signals (UBOs) on magnetic resonance imaging (MRI) and impaired performance on the judgement of line orientation (JLO). Presented at the conjoint meeting of the CNS and ICNA, October 2–8, 1994, San Francisco, CA. Cited in North KN, Riccardi V, Samango-Sprouse C, et al. Cognitive function and academic performance in neurofibromatosis 1: consensus statement from the NF1 Cognitive Disorders Task Force. Neurology 1997;48:1121–1127

23. Moore BD, Slopis JM, Schomer D, Jackson EF, Levy BM. Neuropsychological significance of areas of high signal intensity on brain MRIs of children with neurofibromatosis. Neurology 1996;46:1660–1668

24. Legius E, Descheemaeker MJ, Steyaert J, et al. Neurofibromatosis type 1 in childhood: correlation of MRI findings with intelligence. J Neurol Neurosurg Psychiatry 1995;59:638–640

25. North K, Joy P, Yuille D, Cocks N, Hutchins P. Cognitive function and academic performance in children with neurofibromatosis type 1. Dev Med Child Neurol 1995;37:427–436

26. Legius EM, Descheemaeker MJ, Spaepen A, Casaer P, Fryns JP. Neurofibromatosis type 1 in childhood: a study of the neuropsychological profile in 45 children. Genet Couns 1994;5:51–60

27. Friedman JM, Gutmann DH, MacCollin M, Riccardi VM, eds. Neurofibromatosis: Phenotype, Natural History, and Pathogenesis. 3rd ed. Baltimore: Johns Hopkins University Press; 1999:61

28. American Academy of Pediatrics Committee on Quality Improvement, Subcommittee on Attention-Deficit/Hyperactivity Disorder. Clinical practice guideline: diagnosis and evaluation of the child with attention deficit/hyperactivity disorder. Pediatrics 2000;105:1158–1170

9

Other Features of Neurofibromatosis 1

In addition to the common manifestations of neurofibromatosis 1 (NF1), a variety of seemingly unrelated manifestations are associated with the disorder. These less common but hardly rare manifestations of NF1 may pose significant medical challenges or cause personal discomfort unless diagnosed and managed properly.

◆ Cardiovascular Complications

The body's cardiovascular system consists of the heart and myriad blood vessels that supply nutrients and oxygen to every tissue. NF1 increases the risk of several cardiovascular complications, but it remains unclear why these conditions develop and how they progress naturally over the course of a person's lifetime. Complicating the situation further, it is sometimes difficult to determine which cases of cardiovascular disease arise because of NF1 and which occur coincidentally with the disorder. What is clear is that people with NF bear disproportionately certain types of cardiovascular disease that may contribute to premature mortality in some individuals.

The NF1 Cardiovascular Task Force, an expert panel convened by the National Neurofibromatosis Foundation, sifted through current evidence and concluded that the three most common cardiovascular complications of NF1 are high blood pressure (hypertension), congenital heart disease, and vasculopathy.[1] A brief description of each of these conditions and the panel's recommendation on care is provided below.

Hypertension

Blood pressure is the force of blood as it flows from the heart to the blood vessels, and it is measured in millimeters of mercury (mm Hg). Federal guidelines define normal blood pressure[2] as less than 120/80 mm Hg. The first number is a measure of systolic pressure, when the heart beats, and the second is a measure of diastolic pressure, when the heart relaxes between beats. High blood pressure is defined as 140/90 mm Hg or higher, whereas prehypertension[2] is defined as 120/80 to 139/89 mm Hg. People with higher than normal blood pressure may not be aware of it until it is checked, because often no other symptoms are present. Untreated, however, high blood pressure can cause heart attack, stroke, kidney failure, and other medical problems. In fact, risk of cardiovascular disease doubles with each 20/10 mm Hg increase in blood pressure,[2] starting at 115/75 mm Hg.

Many people with NF1 already have hypertension or are prehypertensive and are at risk of developing high blood pressure as they grow older. High blood pressure can develop in people with NF1 for several reasons. In adults with NF1, the most common type is essential hypertension that develops for no apparent reason and is indistinguishable from that seen in the general population. Several types of secondary hypertension, which arise as a result of another condition or disease, may also occur in people with NF1. When hypertension develops in children and young adults with NF1, particularly in pregnant women, renovascular abnormalities are usually the cause. These abnormalities of blood vessels in the kidneys should be considered a possibility at any age for someone with NF1. In older people tumors known as pheochromocytomas, discussed in Chapter 7, may be the cause. Whenever someone with NF1 develops high blood pressure, it is wise to evaluate all the possible options before making a diagnosis. Treatment depends on the underlying cause.

Essential hypertension in NF1 is probably caused by the same factors that contribute to high blood pressure in the general population. Risk factors include age, excessive weight, diets high in salt, and lack of regular exercise. The current recommendations for target blood pressure for people with NF1 are the same as in the general population. People who have prehypertension should make lifestyle changes to prevent developing high blood pressure. Those who already have hypertension should try to lower their blood pressure readings to less than 140/90 mm Hg. Those who have hypertension and diabetes or chronic kidney disease[2] should aim for less than 130/80 mm Hg.

Lifestyle strategies to reduce blood pressure to healthy levels include weight loss; moderate exercise; a diet that includes more fruits, vegetables, whole grains, and low-fat dairy foods; and reduced intake of alcohol and salt. Several medications are available to reduce high blood pressure in those people who cannot lower it by following diet and exercise regimens. Consult a physician for a personal recommendation.

Renovascular abnormalities occur in ~1 in 100 people with NF1 and include several conditions that can affect blood pressure.[3] The most common is renal artery stenosis, a constriction of one of the major blood vessels that transport blood to the kidneys. When blood flow is reduced, the kidney produces excess amounts of a hormone known as chymosin, triggering the release of other chemicals that raise blood pressure. Less often, an aneurysm—a bulging of a renal blood vessel—may develop in someone with NF1, or other types of abnormalities may develop in blood vessels contained within the kidney itself. To complicate matters, any renovascular abnormality may be part of a more extensive condition known as *vasculopathy,* an impairment of blood vessels that can occur anywhere in the body, usually because a proliferative lesion develops in the artery wall. The exact nature of this lesion and how it arises remain unknown. For instance, people who develop renal artery stenosis are also more likely to suffer from *abdominal aortic coarctation*, a narrowing of the abdominal portion of the body's major blood vessel.

If a renovascular abnormality is suspected, the precise type of disorder can be diagnosed with a combination of blood tests and imaging techniques, such as an ultrasound (which uses sound waves to generate an image), angiography or arteriography (which use radiopaque dyes), and magnetic resonance imaging (MRI, which uses a powerful magnet and computers). The tests ordered depend on the suspected complication. For renal artery stenosis, renal arteriography is the imaging modality of choice, with MRI as an alternative for people who have impaired kidney function or who cannot tolerate arteriography.

Treatment depends on the diagnosis. Some people with NF1 who develop hypertension because of abnormalities in the renal arteries respond to the blood pressure medications described earlier. Others may require surgery. Several surgical options exist for the most common condition, renal artery stenosis. Often the first method used is angioplasty, a procedure in which a balloon-tipped catheter (a flexible narrow tube) is inserted into a narrowed artery. The balloon is then expanded so that the artery widens enough to allow normal blood flow. This procedure is often less successful at treating renal artery stenosis in people with NF1 than the general population.[4] In NF1 the artery may have narrowed because of a proliferative lesion rather than the accumulation of plaque that is more readily cleared by angioplasty. If further treatment is necessary, one option is surgical revascularization, in which blood vessels harvested from somewhere else in the body are grafted onto the kidney to restore blood flow. Another is nephrectomy, removal of the kidney—generally reserved for people with severe disease or those who have failed to respond to other treatments.

Congenital Heart Defects

People with NF1 are more likely than the general population to be born with congenital heart defects. Estimates about the number of people with NF1 who have this condition vary from less than 1% to more than 6%, but the number is probably closer to ~2%.[5] This is at least twice as often as heart defects occur in the general population, where estimates of prevalence vary from 0.4 to 0.9%.[6] Studies in mice suggest that the protein product of the NF1 gene, neurofibromin, is important for prenatal development of the heart, although the precise mechanism remains unknown.[7,8]

Pulmonary stenosis, a constriction of the arteries that pump deoxygenated blood from the heart to the lungs, is the type of congenital heart defect seen most frequently in people with NF1. In this population, this condition accounts for one in four cases of congenital heart disease.[5] Another congenital anomaly of the heart commonly seen in NF1 is coarctation or narrowing of the aorta, the body's largest blood vessel. The aorta transports oxygenated blood from the heart to arteries extending throughout the body.

Diagnosis of a congenital heart defect is made on the basis of physical examination and medical tests. Physical examination of any person diagnosed with NF1 should include a careful assessment of heart function, including blood pressure reading and auscultation, the use of a stethoscope to hear sounds made by the heart. If a heart murmur is detected, the patient should be referred to a cardiologist for further evaluation and testing, including an echocardiogram. This test uses sound waves to provide a picture of the heart as it beats as well as information about valve function and muscle health. This helps to determine whether the abnormality is pulmonary stenosis, aortic coarctation, or another type of heart defect. When aortic coarctation is suspected, blood pressure measurements should be taken in all four extremities (arms and legs) to determine the extent and effect of the narrowed aorta. Further evaluation and treatment options depend on the defect and age of the person.

Vasculopathy

The vascular system consists of blood vessels that help oxygenated blood circulate throughout the body and then return to the heart for reoxygenation. In some people with NF1, blood vessels may become constricted, blocked, or damaged—a condition known as vasculopathy. These events may occur in any blood vessel, and usually multiple blood vessels are involved. The changes include narrowing (stenosis), blockage (occlusion), or a circumscribed bulging of a blood vessel (aneurysm). In rare but severe cases, a vessel may rupture, causing internal hemorrhage. Most people with NF1 who have vasculopathy do not experience symptoms; for that reason, it is unclear how many people with the disorder have this complication. Symptoms are most likely to develop in people with renal artery abnormalities or cerebrovascular abnormalities of blood vessels in the brain.

Cerebrovascular anomalies are not common in people with NF1. When they do occur, most often the carotid artery, a major blood vessel at the base of the brain, is narrowed or obstructed. Smaller vessels will sprout around the blocked artery as the body seeks to compensate for the sudden reduction of blood flow to the area, creating a condition known as "moyamoya" (Fig. 9–1). Moyamoya is more common in children with NF1 who undergo cranial radiation for treatment of a brain tumor because radiation can damage blood vessels. Surgical procedures to redirect blood flow around the obstruction are available to individuals with moyamoya.

Other types of cerebrovascular abnormalities include aneurysms and malformation of blood vessels in the brain.

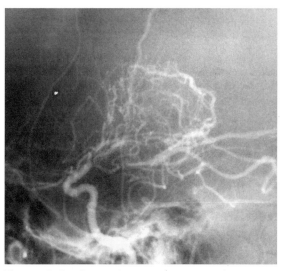

Figure 9–1   An angiogram demonstrating moya-moya syndrome in a child with NF1. The condition occurs when a blood vessel becomes blocked and smaller collateral blood vessels form in the surrounding area.

Cerebrovascular irregularities can occur at any time in someone with NF1. Typical symptoms include weakness, headaches, seizures, and involuntary movements. In children, this usually results from ischemia, death of brain tissue due to cessation of blood flow to part of the brain. In adults, the same symptoms may indicate an internal hemorrhage caused by blood vessel rupture. Any person with NF1 who suddenly develops a neurological deficit should be evaluated promptly, for this may indicate the existence of a blood clot (thrombus) or obstruction. Diagnosis of these events is based on physical examination and brain imaging tests. MRI is usually ordered first, sometimes followed by cerebral angiography. Because some of the symptoms associated with cerebrovascular malfunction may have another cause, the individual should be evaluated for a heart attack or stroke.

If a cerebrovascular abnormality is detected, treatment is the same as in the general population. An initial strategy may include medications such as aspirin and blood thinners to prevent blood clots from forming in narrowed arteries. In other cases brain surgery may be necessary to remove obstructions or prevent vessels from rupturing.

◆ Orthopedic Manifestations

NF1 may alter height and bone development in a variety of ways. It is unclear why. Fortunately, when orthopedic involvement occurs, early detection can prevent or minimize functional impairment and skeletal deformity. Severe skeletal deformities are rare, although they are often the ones that are pictured in medical textbooks. Because signs of orthopedic changes may be subtle at first, a child diagnosed with NF1 should receive regular orthopedic examinations until early adulthood (see Chapter 5). The most frequent types of skeletal manifestations associated with NF1 are described briefly below.

Spinal Problems

The spinal column (Fig. **9–2**) consists of 33 bones called vertebrae that extend from the base of the skull to the pelvis. The spine surrounds and protects the spinal cord, the network of nerves that connect the brain to the peripheral nervous system. Each peripheral nerve is rooted in the spinal cord and then extends a series of nerve branches outward to locations throughout the body. The cervical section is the topmost portion of the spine; the thoracic section is located at the rear wall of the chest and attached to the ribs; the lumbar section constitutes the lower back; the

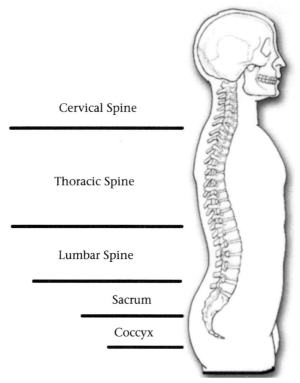

Cervical Spine

Thoracic Spine

Lumbar Spine

Sacrum

Coccyx

Figure 9–2   The regions of the spine. (Courtesy of Harriet Greenfield, with permission.)

sacrum and coccyx consist of fused vertebrae in the pelvic area. NF1 can deform the spine in several ways.

Scoliosis

Curvature of the spine is the most common type of spinal distortion seen in people with NF1. A healthy spine, viewed from behind, runs straight up the middle of the back dividing the trunk into halves. In scoliosis, the spine curves and distorts the normal symmetry of the trunk. Depending on the severity of the curve, other abnormalities may be evident, such as uneven shoulder height, a pronounced pelvic tilt, or a larger space between arm and trunk on one side of the body when a person is standing. It is not known what causes scoliosis in people with NF1, just as it is not known what causes most cases in the general population. Contrary to what some people believe, scoliosis does not result from poor posture, back strain, or active sports.

Scoliosis is found in less than 1% of men and ~2% of women in the general population,[9] but in people with NF1, it presents in 10%.[10(p262)] Children with NF1 tend to develop scoliosis earlier than other children, usually by 10 years of age,[11] underscoring the need for regular physical examinations. Sometimes scoliosis is so mild that it does not require treatment. To prevent potentially serious developments, however, any child with NF1 should be examined for scoliosis annually as part of a comprehensive physical examination (see Chapter 5). Once scoliosis is diagnosed, the child should be reexamined regularly to determine whether the curve is progressing.

The most common type of scoliosis in NF1 involves a type of curve indistinguishable from that seen in the general population: a gentle lateral curve in the shape of a C that involves about one third of the spine (Fig. **9–3**). Any portion of the spine may be susceptible, although people with NF1 often develop a curvature in the lower cervical and upper thoracic spine, sometimes accompanied by *kyphosis*, a hump. Management of this type of scoliosis is similar to that in the general population and depends on a combination of factors: the degree of curvature, its location

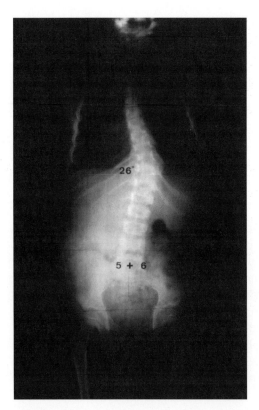

Figure 9–3 This radiograph shows a long C-shaped curvature of the spine in a $5\frac{1}{2}$-year-old child with NF1. Although this type of scoliosis is also seen in the general population, usually beginning during adolescence, children with NF1 tend to develop these curves much earlier.

and rate of progression, and the age of the child. Curves located in the thoracic portion of the spine are more likely to progress than are lumbar curves. Because a curve is most likely to progress while the child is actively growing, any curve that is already significant before adolescence may progress further during the growth spurts associated with puberty. Management options for this most common form of scoliosis in NF1 are many, but generally fall into three broad categories: monitoring without intervention, bracing, or surgery.

Monitoring without intervention is appropriate when scoliosis is first diagnosed, and in anyone who has reached skeletal maturity and has a curve less than 40 degrees in magnitude.[9]

Bracing is generally recommended for children and adolescents with spinal curves that are 25 to 40 degrees in magnitude,[12] are actively progressing, or are expected to progress because of the child's age or the curve's location. A brace, known as an orthosis, comes in various types and materials, and the exact prescription depends on an orthopedist's advice. In general, braces used to treat scoliosis are hard and resemble vests (Fig. **9–4**). The device is worn for a significant part of each day (16 to

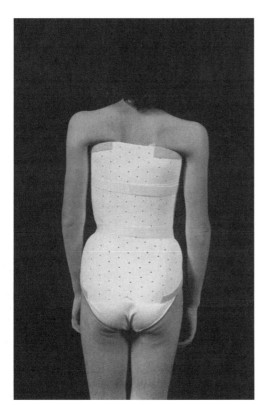

Figure 9–4 A lightweight orthosis worn underneath the patient's clothing may be used to treat mild scoliosis or to prevent curve progression while the child continues to grow.

23 hours). Although it can be worn under the child's usual clothing, braces do tend to be uncomfortable, hot, and cumbersome—all of which make them unpleasant for most children and adolescents. In some instances, braces are effective in stopping a curve from progressing further, but many children with NF1 have spines with such sharp angles that surgery may be necessary.

Surgery is usually reserved as an option of last resort because of the inherent risks. Recommendations vary, but generally surgery becomes an option when a curve has progressed to 50 degrees in magnitude, or where the curve has progressed significantly in spite of bracing.[12] Some orthopedic surgeons recommend treatment even earlier, when the curve is 40 or 45 degrees in magnitude.[9] Surgery is beneficial in that it can help to correct the curve and reduce or eliminate any related deformity. The exact procedure recommended depends on the location and degree of curve. A common procedure for curves in the thoracic area of the spine is known as posterior spinal fusion. Individual vertebrae in the spinal column are fused together so that the curve is eliminated or significantly reduced. Metal rods and wire are permanently attached to the back of the vertebrae to help support the healing spine. Spinal fusion limits mobility, but it prevents nerve damage, deformity, and even potentially life-threatening complications of the lung or heart in people with rapidly progressing or severe curves. Other surgical procedures may be recommended, including less invasive endoscopic surgery (done through small incisions). Because surgical techniques and instrumentation have advanced, most people do not require postoperative casts or braces, and they return home within a week after surgery. Some physical therapy to regain mobility may be required.

Dystrophic Scoliosis

This type of scoliosis is less common in people with NF1 but potentially far more serious. It alters only a small number of vertebrae, resulting in a sharp, angular curve (Fig. **9–5**), and is usually seen only in people with NF1. This form of curvature begins early in life, most often between 6 and 10 years of age,[10(p263)] and progresses within a matter of months rather than years. Treatment for dystrophic scoliosis generally leads to surgery, even if bracing is tried first.

Other Spinal Manifestations

Additional spinal manifestations associated with NF1 include erosion of vertebrae by neurofibromas, kyphosis, and scalloping, a rippling wave-like pattern on the surface of vertebrae. These conditions may occur on their own or in conjunction with scoliosis.

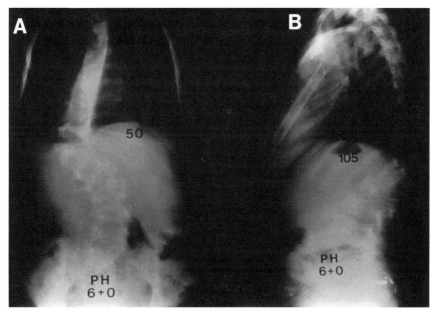

Figure 9–5   A: This radiograph shows the sharp, angular type of scoliosis (dystrophic) that is found almost exclusively in patients with NF1. Although only a relatively small area of the spine is involved, surgical treatment is usually necessary to avoid severe deformity. B: In the same patient the lateral curvature, or scoliosis, is complicated by a front-to-back curvature known as kyphosis.

Destruction of vertebrae by spinal neurofibromas is an unusual but serious complication of NF1. This process begins when neurofibromas grow along the roots of peripheral nerves, which are located within the vertebrae. Should spinal neurofibromas grow excessively, they can erode individual vertebrae, compress the spinal cord, and interfere with nerve function. This can cause pain and weakness or loss of function in arms, legs, or other parts of the body, depending on the nerve location. Spinal surgery is an option, but the benefits in gain of function or lessening of pain must be weighed against risk, which might include loss of function and even paralysis.

Vertebral scalloping is probably more common than realized, but it causes no physical symptoms and may not be detected unless an x-ray is taken of the spine. The back or *dorsal* surface of vertebrae in the lumbar section of the spine is the usual location.

Kyphosis is a condition in which the spine curves outward into a hump or gradually rounded back. Cervical kyphosis, occurring in the top-most area of the spine, is a common complication of dystrophic scoliosis. The curvature usually develops slowly and does not cause pain at first;

thus, it is important to watch for in people with NF1 and dystrophic scoliosis. A neck brace may help to prevent further progression. If not,
surgery to fuse cervical vertebrae may be necessary. It is risky to allow
cervical kyphosis to progress because the curvature may place pressure on
the spinal cord, compromising nerve function and even interfering with
vital functions such as breathing.

Additional Orthopedic Problems

Short Stature

Individuals with NF1 may be tall or short. As in the general population,
there is a great variation in height. When the *average* height for people
with NF1 is compared with that of the general population, however,
people with NF1 tend to be shorter than unaffected people of the same
age and sex. About 80% of people with NF1 are shorter than
average.[10(p282)] One group of researchers studying a representative sampling of people with NF1 concluded that the average height for people
with the disorder consistently falls below the 25th percentile on standard growth charts.[10(p253)] This means that 75% of the general population
is taller than the average person with NF1, and 25% are shorter. One in
three people with NF1 are significantly shorter, falling below the 5th
percentile.[10(p253)] This means that 95% of the general population is taller.
If a child with NF1 is shorter than average, this characteristic will be evident from childhood through early adulthood. These findings apply to
both males and females.

It is not clear why people with NF1 may be shorter than siblings and
other peers, and why only some people with the disorder exhibit this
manifestation. People with NF1 who are short do not suffer from deficien-
cies of growth hormones, hypothalamic or pituitary gland lesions, or any
specific bone ailments. Short stature causes no physical complications.

Abnormal Bone Development

Bone dysplasia occurs in ~14% of people with NF1 and usually is detected
in the first year of life.[13] The most common bone abnormalities seen in
NF1 include dysplastic vertebrae (discussed earlier), limb abnormalities,
and a distinctive craniofacial dysplasia involving the sphenoid wing, a
bone at the base of the skull that helps form portions of the eye and nasal
cavities.

In most cases, sphenoid wing dysplasia (Fig. **9–6**) causes no physical
effects and may manifest only as a subtle asymmetry of the skull. Occasionally, in a severe instance, the eye socket becomes deformed and
reconstructive surgery may be required.

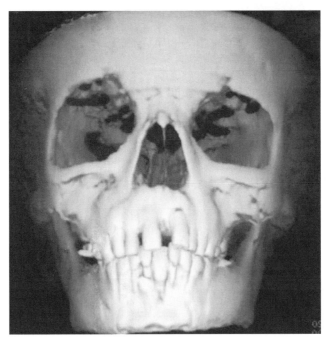

Figure 9–6   Sphenoid dysplasia is usually unilateral; in this case, it enlarges the right orbit (seen on the left side in this figure).

A concave chest, known medically as pectus excavatum, may be present in individuals with NF1. In some cases, the effect is so mild it is hardly noticeable; in other cases, it is severe enough that a significant indentation is visible on the chest area. The breastbone (sternum) and ribs may be included. It is not known what causes the concave chest and the condition poses no medical challenge.

The long bones of the body include the collarbone (clavicle) and those in the arms and legs. Any of these bones may become deformed in NF1, although it is not yet clear what biological mechanism is involved. Sometimes the bone curves outward. Such bowing may be subtle at first, especially in the first months or years of life. In most cases, only one bone is bowed. The difference becomes apparent as a subtle asymmetry that may become more noticeable in time as the child grows. Most often it is the shinbone (tibia) that tends to bow in an anterolateral direction, which means that the lower part of the leg is curved forward and to the outer side (Figs. **9–7** and **9–8**). The thighbone (femur), forearm bones (radius and ulna), and clavicle may also curve outward. Mild bowing can be treated with orthoses, flexible or rigid supports that are wrapped around

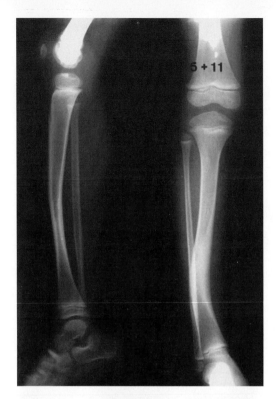

Figure 9–7 These radiographs show anterolateral bowing of the tibia in a 5-year, 11-month-old boy with NF1.

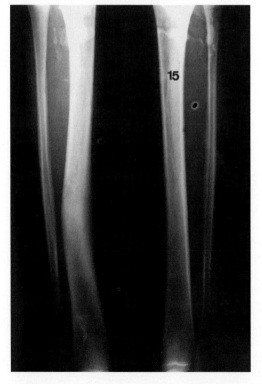

Figure 9–8 Following the use of orthoses during growth, the deformity has improved and the bones are much stronger at 15 years of age.

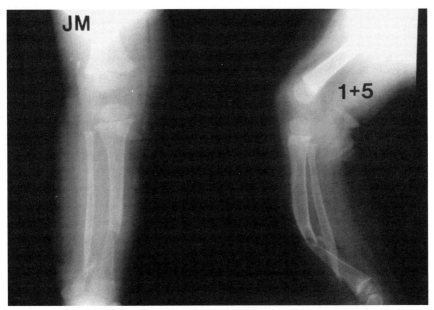

Figure 9–9   Fractures of the tibia in young patients with NF1 often fail to heal. This condition, known as pseudarthrosis, may be seen in these radiographs of a 17-month-old child.

the limb to support the bone as the child grows. In more severe cases, the bone may fracture and the child may require orthopedic surgery.

Pseudarthrosis, or "false joint," occurs when a bone fractures and does not heal properly, or when bowing becomes so extreme that it causes a severe angling in the bone (Fig. **9–9**). This happens most often in the weight-bearing bones, especially the tibia. A cast to heal the fracture may be tried first, but this method is usually not successful. Several surgical options exist, including grafting of bone tissue harvested from the other leg or hip, sometimes accompanied by the insertion of a metal pin or the application of an electrical current to help the bone heal. Unfortunately, these procedures are not always effective once a break has occurred. Some children go through one surgical procedure after another, with poor results, and must have the leg amputated. Although brutal to contemplate, leg amputation often leads to a better quality of life for some children.

Bone overgrowth is another potential complication of NF1 and bones in the legs are usual sites (Fig. **9–10**). The bone grows longer and thicker on one side of the body than on the other. The result is a noticeable asymmetry in the limbs, which interferes with movement if not treated. In most cases, surgeons destroy growth plates, or physes, in the bone that is overgrown; these structures direct the rate of growth in that limb and

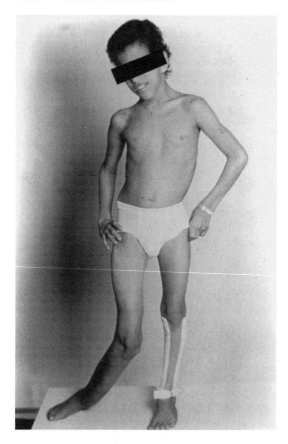

Figure 9–10 Overgrowth of the long bones, as seen in this patient, may result from disturbances to the physes, or growth plates, by neurofibromas.

may behave abnormally because of pressure by neurofibromas. The corrective procedure, known as epiphysiodesis, must be timed precisely so that the other limb can continue to grow until it matches the overgrown limb in length and size.

Another type of bone dysplasia involves thinning of the long bones, quite frequently the tibia (Fig. **9–11**). Thinning may occur in any bone in the body. Children with thinning of the long bones are prone to fractures. In most cases, an orthosis or brace will sufficiently protect and support the fragile bone.

Additional Skeletal Problems

Bone deformity may also occur as a consequence of aggressive growth of plexiform neurofibromas. An adjacent bone may be eroded by a growing neurofibroma or grow excessively around the tumor, resulting in deformity. It is not known why bones are sometimes altered by neurofibroma growth,

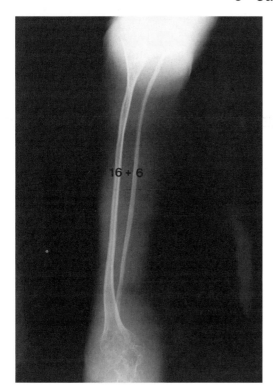

Figure 9–11 This radiograph shows very thin bones in the lower part of the leg that require bracing and careful observation to avoid fracture and progressive deformity in this area.

but the changes probably reflect some combination of mechanical pressure caused by the expanding tumor, invasion of bone by neurofibroma cells, altered muscle support, and abnormalities in blood vessels that supply bone tissue with nutrients. Surgery can correct severe deformities.

◆ Endocrine System Abnormalities

The endocrine system consists of glands located throughout the body that secrete hormones, chemical messengers that regulate growth and development, sexual and reproductive functions, metabolism, and mood, among other functions. Several types of endocrine system abnormalities occur in NF1, although they are not common.

Early or Delayed Puberty

Although most adolescents with NF1 experience normal puberty, ~1 to 4% experience it earlier or later than normal.[14,15] Puberty is a process that usually takes about 4 to 5 years to complete, starting between ages 8 and 13 in girls, and 9 and 14 in boys.[16] A wide variety in ages of onset and rates of progression in puberty is considered to be normal. Biochemically, puberty is initiated when the hypothalamus in the brain releases gonadotropin-releasing hormone. This stimulates the release of two hormones from the pituitary gland, a small gland located just beneath the brain, that in turn stimulate the production of estrogen and progesterone in the ovaries and testosterone in the testes. The first physical signs of puberty are the development of breasts and pubic hair in girls, testicular enlargement and pubic hair in boys, and growth spurts in both sexes. As puberty progresses, girls start to menstruate and boys develop facial hair and deeper voices.

Precocious puberty occurs when the physical or hormonal signs of puberty occur in boys younger than 9, in white girls younger than 7, and in black girls younger than 6 years old.[17] In children with NF1, precocious puberty is usually caused by an optic glioma placing pressure on the hypothalamus and stimulating a cascade of hormones earlier than is normal. Any child with NF1 who has an optic glioma, therefore, should be monitored for precocious puberty (see Chapter 7).

Diagnosis should include annual height and weight measurements, to determine whether a growth spurt has started, and medical history and physical examination to detect the first outward manifestations of puberty. In girls, breast enlargement begins subtly with the appearance of breast buds that may occur on one side first and are sometimes hard to distinguish from fat. Physicians can more readily tell the difference by having the child lie down during the examination. In both boys and girls, growth of pubic hair may be subtle at first, but a physician can determine whether genital changes such as enlargement of the clitoris and testicles have begun. These changes precede by one or more years the more obvious manifestations of puberty, menstruation, and penis growth. If early puberty is suspected, the physician may recommend blood and other laboratory tests to measure hormone levels to confirm a diagnosis. Sometimes x-rays are also ordered, to compare the maturational age of a child's bones to his or her chronological age.

Precocious puberty poses two major issues, one psychological and the other physical. Children who develop faster than peers may be embarrassed by the physical changes they experience, be subjected to teasing, and act out or behave differently. Children who undergo precocious puberty tend to be taller than peers initially but ultimately may not achieve the same height as siblings or parents, mainly because puberty encourages skeletal maturation that slows growth.

Management of precocious puberty in children with NF1 generally involves hormone therapy, sometimes combined with chemotherapy depending on the size and rate of growth of the optic glioma. The medications most often used are gonadotropin-releasing hormone (GnRH) agonists, which suppress the production of sex hormones by the pituitary gland. These medications halt puberty for as long as they are taken, slowing the rate of bone maturity. GnRH agonists must be injected; some are given daily whereas others may be given every 3 to 4 weeks. Side effects are usually mild and temporary. Once a child is placed on hormone therapy, follow-up visits should occur every 3 months to gauge results and monitor hormone levels.[16]

Delayed puberty sometimes occurs in NF1, although it is not clear why. Puberty is considered delayed when it begins after age 13 in girls and after 14 in boys. Diagnosis involves the same process described above for precocious puberty, except that blood tests may also be analyzed for conditions such as anemia and diabetes, which can delay puberty. Sometimes a tendency to late puberty is inherited and no treatment is necessary. In other cases, delayed puberty may be caused by damage to the hypothalamus or pituitary gland, possibly by tumors associated with NF1. Treatment usually involves hormone therapy to stimulate puberty and surgery if necessary.

◆ Additional Challenges in Neurofibromatosis 1

Fertility and Pregnancy

Fertility

Men and women with NF1 are just as fertile as people in the general population. They tend to have fewer children, however, either because of lifestyle choices or concern about passing the disorder on to offspring.

It is unknown what effect oral contraceptives have on manifestations of NF1. Some women have found that dermal neurofibromas have increased in size or number while they were taking birth control pills, but the evidence so far is anecdotal. More research needs to be done about the effects of hormones on NF1 manifestations.

Pregnancy

Most women with NF1 who decide to bear children experience normal pregnancies and deliveries. There are exceptions, however. Women who have large pelvic or genital neurofibromas may not be able to deliver the child vaginally and instead undergo a cesarean delivery. Pregnancy may also worsen some manifestations of NF1, although this does not happen to every woman with the disorder. Hormonal fluctuations have long been suspected of stimulating neurofibroma growth. This theory was bolstered by a recent report showing that some neurofibromas are sensitive to progesterone, a hormone that is elevated during pregnancy (see Chapter 6). Although no consensus about cause has been established, some women may find that existing dermal neurofibromas may gradually grow markedly larger and inflamed during pregnancy; within weeks after delivery, they tend to return to prepregnancy size.[10(p60)] New dermal neurofibromas may emerge, especially during the third trimester, and these will remain after delivery. Diffuse plexiform neurofibromas sometimes start to grow again during pregnancy, but they may regress partially or fully within several weeks of delivery.[10(p60)] These tumors may turn malignant during pregnancy in some patients. Women and their physicians, therefore, should be familiar with the signs and symptoms of malignancy (see Chapter 6).

Women with NF1 who become pregnant may develop high blood pressure because of a previously unrecognized renovascular abnormality, or experience exacerbated symptoms if they already have essential hypertension. Whatever the cause, high blood pressure during pregnancy needs to be monitored. Although many women deliver healthy babies in spite of high blood pressure during pregnancy, hypertension can harm the mother's internal organs and sometimes results in early delivery and low birth weight for the baby. In severe cases, the pregnant woman may develop preeclampsia, a life-threatening condition for both mother and developing child.

In many cases, the lifestyle changes described earlier in this chapter, such as reducing salt consumption, making other dietary changes, and increasing physical activity, may help to reduce blood pressure sufficiently during pregnancy. If a woman is already taking medication to control blood pressure, it is possible she may be able to continue taking it, lower the dose, or change to a different type of drug. To avoid any harm to the developing fetus, this issue should be discussed carefully with a physician.

Chronic Itching

A constant itching sensation, known medically as pruritus, has been associated with NF1. It also occurs in the general population. Sometimes it is restricted to only one or a few parts of the body; at other times the sensation occurs all over. Many people find pruritus as uncomfortable and distracting as pain. It is not entirely clear why NF1 causes itching in some people. It is known that histamine, a substance produced naturally in the body, can cause itching when injected into the skin. When mast cells in the skin are injured, they release histamine. One theory is that when mast cells overproliferate, as they do in neurofibromas, the resulting release of histamine may cause an itch. Common antihistamines may help to relieve symptoms.

Pruritus occasionally occurs because of infection or an undiagnosed cancer. Anyone who experiences this symptom should consult a physician to determine the underlying cause and have it treated. Antibiotics, for instance, eliminate itching that is caused by an infection. Medications are also available to treat some of the itching associated with cancers and their treatment. Most cases of pruritus arise for no apparent reason, and a management strategy usually develops through trial and error by the concerned individual. Some common strategies to relieve itching are listed below.

Lifestyle Changes

◆ **Interrupt the Itch Cycle**   When an itch is scratched, the area sometimes becomes more itchy. To break this cycle, apply a cool cloth or ice pack to the area.

◆ **Choose Mild Soaps**   Some soaps contain harsh detergents that aggravate or dry skin. Experiment with soaps to find mild products.

◆ **Moisturize**   Dry skin may itch. Moisturizers lubricate the skin and coat the surface with a thin film that encourages continued moisture production. Ingredients vary, and some experimentation may be necessary to find the product that works best.

◆ **Warm Baths and Soaks**   Some people find that soaking the troublesome area of skin in warm water once a day helps to relieve itching. Hot water may exacerbate itching, however, as does soaking more than once a day or longer than 30 minutes. Some people add oil to the warm water to soothe the skin.

◆ **Adjust Room Temperature**   Itching is aggravated by air that is hot or low in humidity. Keeping rooms cool and adding a humidifier may help.

◆ **Choose Proper Clothing**   Loose-fitting, lightweight, cotton clothes alleviate itching in some people who are sensitive to wool and synthetic fabrics.

◆ **Eliminate Detergent Residue**   Many detergents and fabric softeners leave a residue on clothing after washing, and this exacerbates itching in some people. Add one teaspoon of vinegar per quart of water during the rinse cycle, or purchase detergent for baby clothes.

◆ **Distractions**   Some people find that listening to music, doing imagery exercises, or massaging another part of the body help distract them so that the itching feels less intense.

Medication strategies include several drugs that work in different ways. Consult a physician for a personal recommendation.

◆ Constipation and Gastrointestinal Distress

Some people with NF1 experience frequent stomachaches, abdominal pain, and chronic constipation—either alone or in combination. It is not clear why. One possibility is that neurofibromas in the intestines may interfere with digestion. In many cases, however, gastrointestinal distress may develop for the same reasons as in the general population, including food allergies, overall diet, medication use, and changes in the environment. If these conditions persist and are bothersome, consult a physician to determine the cause and obtain recommendations for treatment.

Chronic constipation is the most frequent type of gastrointestinal aberration reported by people with NF1. This may manifest as a decrease in bowel movements or difficulty and straining in having one. Seek medical advice immediately if blood is present in the stool, which may be a sign of colorectal cancer, or if constipation persists for more than 3 weeks after trying dietary and lifestyle changes. Chronic constipation may create other problems, such as hemorrhoids that develop from repeated straining, or spot bleeding caused by hard stools that tear the skin.

Diagnosis is usually made on the basis of medical history and physical examination. A physician will ask about symptoms, onset, and duration. A digital rectal exam helps to assess the tone of the anal sphincter, the muscle that closes off the anus, as well as determine the presence of any blood, obstruction, or sensitivity in the area. Only in severe cases do patients need tests such as barium enema, sigmoidoscopy, or colonoscopy, which assess intestinal health in various ways.

Management strategies vary. Most cases of constipation in NF1 can be alleviated by making one or more of the following lifestyle changes:

◆ **Increase Intake of Dietary Fiber and Fluids**   Dietary fiber is found in whole grain foods, fruits, and vegetables. Fiber supplements are also available. Aim for 20 to 35 g of fiber each day. Fiber helps alleviate constipation because it is not digested and it absorbs water as it moves through the digestive tract, which softens the stool and makes bowel movements easier. It is important to drink enough fluids to help the body adjust to increased fiber intake, however. Otherwise the result may be gastrointestinal distress. Drink at least eight 8-ounce glasses of water or uncaffeinated beverages per day. Caffeine, a diuretic, causes the body to lose water.

◆ **Exercise Daily**   Moderate exercise can help to alleviate constipation in some people. It is not clear why.

◆ **Become a Creature of Habit**   Having a bowel movement at the same time every day helps some people, perhaps by acclimating the body.

Laxatives and suppositories are recommended only when lifestyle changes fail to make a difference. These should be viewed as temporary measures, because some are harmful or habit forming when used for too long.

◆ The Personal Perspective

Nancy B.: "In some cases of NF1, the sphenoid bone doesn't properly fuse. So I have a hole in my skull. It's elliptical in shape, about 2 inches by 1 inch and located on one side of my head. The same doctor who originally diagnosed my NF said that if I were a professional hockey player, he'd recommend that I have a protective plate inserted, but otherwise not to worry, so I haven't."

Angela W.: "I did have some neurofibroma growth during pregnancy. A lot of them popped up on my hand and one on my chin. But that's it. I was very fortunate. I did have a little high blood pressure at the end, but that was probably nerves."

References

1. Friedman JM, Arbiser J, Epstein JA, et al. Cardiovascular disease in neurofibromatosis 1: report of the NF1 Cardiovascular Task Force. Genet Med 2002;4:105–111
2. Chobanian AM, Bakris GL, Black HR, et al. The seventh report of the Joint National Committee on Prevention, Detection, Evaluation, and Treatment of High Blood Pressure. JAMA 2003; 289:2560–2571
3. Finley JL, Dabbs DJ. Renal vascular smooth muscle proliferation in neurofibromatosis. Hum Pathol 1988;19: 107–110
4. Fossali E, Minoja M, Intermite R, Spreafico C, Casalini E, Serini F. Percutaneous transluminal renal angioplasty in neurofibromatosis. Pediatr Nephrol 1995;9:623–625
5. Lin AE, Birch PH, Korf BR, et al. Cardiovascular malformations and other cardiac abnormalities in neurofibromatosis 1. Am J Med Genet 2000;95: 108–117
6. Hoffman JL. Congenital heart disease: incidence and inheritance. Pediatr Clin North Am 1990;37:25–43
7. Brannan CI, Perkins AS, Vogel KS, et al. Targeted disruption of the neurofibromatosis type 1 gene leads to developmental abnormalities in heart and various neural crest-derived tissues. Genes Dev 1994;8:1019–1029

8. Jacks T, Shih TS, Schmitt EM, Bronson RT, Bernards A, Weinberg RA. Tumour predisposition in mice heterozygous for a targeted mutation in *NF1*. Nat Genet 1994;7:353–361

9. Scoliosis treatment. Scoliosis Research Institute Web site. Available at: *http://www.scoliosisrx.com*

10. Friedman JM, Gutmann DH, MacCollin M, Riccardi VM, eds. Neurofibromatosis: Phenotype, Natural History, and Pathogenesis. 3rd ed. Baltimore: Johns Hopkins University Press; 1999

11. Rubenstein AE, Korf BR. Neurofibromatosis: A Handbook for Patients, Families, and Health-Care Professionals. New York: Thieme Medical Publishers; 1990:126

12. In-depth review of scoliosis: treatment of adolescent idiopathic scoliosis. Scoliosis Research Society Web site. Available at: http://www.srs.org/htm/library/review/review06.htm.

13. DeBella K, Szudek J, Friedman JM. Use of the National Institutes of Health criteria for diagnosis of neurofibromatosis 1 in children. Pediatrics 2000;105:608–614

14. Riccardi VM. Neurofibromatosis: Phenotype, Natural History, and Pathogenesis. 2nd ed. Baltimore: Johns Hopkins University Press; 1992. Cited in Friedman JM, Gutmann DH, MacCollin M, Riccardi VM, eds. Neurofibromatosis: Phenotype, Natural History, and Pathogenesis. 3rd ed. Baltimore: Johns Hopkins University Press; 1999:283

15. Friedman JM, Birch PH. Type 1 neurofibromatosis: a descriptive analysis of the disorder in 1,728 patients. Am J Med Genet 1997;70:138–143

16. Precocious puberty. The MAGIC Foundation for Children's Growth Web site. Available at: http://www.magicfoundation.org/print/cppp.html.

17. Kaplowitz PB. Precocious puberty. eMedicine [serial online]. January 17, 2002. Available at: http://www.emedicine.com/ped/topic1882.htm.

10

Diagnosis and Overall Management of Neurofibromatosis 2

The hallmark feature of neurofibromatosis 2 (NF2) is a slow-growing tumor on the eighth cranial nerve in both ears. This nerve has two branches. The acoustic nerve enables people to hear by transmitting sound sensation to the brain. The vestibular nerve function is related to balance. The tumors are known as vestibular schwannomas because they originate in Schwann cells that help to form the myelin sheath around nerves in the central nervous system.

People with NF2 are at increased risk of developing other types of nervous system tumors as well. These include spinal schwannomas that tend to grow within the spinal cord and between the vertebrae. People with NF2 may also develop ependymomas and *meningiomas*, tumors that grow along the membranes covering the brain and spinal cord. Others may develop a typical type of *cataract* (juvenile posterior subcapsular lenticular opacity) or, more rarely, orbital meningiomas. These typical features of NF2 are discussed in detail later in this chapter.

The current diagnostic criteria for NF2 are listed in Table **10–1**. These criteria are based on those originally developed in the same 1987 National Institutes of Health (NIH) Consensus Conference that established criteria for an NF1 diagnosis,[1] which, in 1990, were updated.[2] The original criteria establish bilateral tumors of the eighth cranial (auditory) nerve as a hallmark feature of NF2. Additional criteria were proposed by Evans and colleagues[3] in 1992 so that physicians could recognize rare cases of NF2

Table 10–1   Diagnostic Criteria for Neurofibromatosis 2 (NF2)

Individuals with the Following Clinical Features Have Confirmed (Definite) NF2	Individuals with the Following Clinical Features Should Be Evaluated for NF2 (Presumptive or Probable NF2)
Bilateral vestibular schwannomas *or* Family history of NF2 (first-degree relative) *plus* Unilateral vestibular schwannoma before age 30 *or* Any two of the following: • Meningioma • Glioma • Schwannoma • Juvenile posterior subcapsular lenticular opacities/juvenile cortical cataract	Unilateral vestibular schwannoma before age 30 *plus* at least one of the following: • Meningioma • Glioma • Schwannoma • Juvenile posterior subcapsular lenticular opacities/juvenile cortical cataract Multiple meningiomas (two or more) *plus* unilateral vestibular schwannomas before age 30 *or* one of the following: • Glioma • Schwannoma • Juvenile posterior subcapsular lenticular opacities/juvenile cortical cataract

Adapted from Gutmann DH, Aylsworth A, Carey JC, et al. The diagnostic evaluation and multidisciplinary management of neurofibromatosis 1 and neurofibromatosis 2. JAMA 1997;278:54, with permission.

that do not present the hallmark feature of bilateral tumors of the eighth cranial nerve. The most current criteria are those established by the Clinical Care Advisory Board of the National Neurofibromatosis Foundation, which, in 1997, proposed further refinements of the diagnostic criteria.[4]

First, the NF Foundation committee recommended that the hallmark feature, bilateral eighth-nerve masses, be described as "bilateral vestibular schwannomas," to reflect advancements in knowledge about the pathology and origin of these tumors. The committee also sought to make the diagnostic criteria more flexible, so that physicians could distinguish between people who definitely have NF2 (whose manifestations match the NIH criteria) and those who might have the disorder because their manifestations more closely match the Evans criteria. To accomplish this, the committee proposed a new category of manifestations that provide a "presumptive" diagnosis of NF2.

Studies have shown that NF2 is typically diagnosed several, and in some cases many, years after onset of symptoms, underscoring the need to screen and monitor those at risk because of a family history of the disorder.

In most cases, physicians can diagnose NF2 on the basis of the consensus criteria described in Table **10–1**. Diagnosis of NF2 is straightforward in individuals who have bilateral vestibular schwannomas, tumors located on the eighth cranial nerve leading from the inner ear to the brain, causing changes in balance and hearing. A diagnosis may be more challenging in two groups of people: individuals with a family history of the disorder who do not yet show manifestations, and individuals with no family history who develop one or more manifestations suggestive of the disorder but who do not yet have bilateral vestibular schwannomas. Both groups should be considered at risk for NF2 and undergo follow-up evaluations until a diagnosis can be confirmed or ruled out.

Given the complexities and rarity of NF2, if the disorder is suspected, an individual should be referred to a specialty treatment center for diagnosis, evaluation, and treatment. These centers not only have physicians and staff who are experienced in managing NF2, but also use teams of specialists to manage the disorder.

◆ Natural History of Neurofibromatosis 2

Because NF2 is so rare, few studies have been done about the development and natural progression of the disorder over the life span. Clinical experience indicates, however, that the course of NF2 varies greatly in the population but tends to be more or less the same within a given family. Although diagnosis of NF2 usually takes place in adulthood, signs of the disease may be present in childhood but are so subtle that they are missed, particularly in children without a family history of the disorder. In fact, studies of the natural history of NF2 have reported a consistent and significant delay between onset of symptoms and accurate diagnosis, emphasizing the need for better surveillance, especially for children with a family history of the disorder.

Typically, symptoms of NF2 are first noticed between 18 and 22 years of age,[3,5] although one in 10 people with the disorder will become symptomatic before they are 10 years old.[4(p55)] In some unusual individuals symptoms first appear after 35 years of age.[6(p304)] The most frequent presenting symptom is hearing loss and/or ringing in the ears *(tinnitus)*. Less often a visit to the doctor is prompted by changes in balance sensory powers, or vision, or by limb weakness, seizures, skin tumors.[3,5] In children suspected of having NF2 because of a family history of the disorder, the first manifestations may be a posterior capsular opacity or a skin schwannoma.

NF2 is a progressive disorder, but the rate of progression varies greatly, perhaps because of the influence of other genes and biological factors as yet unknown. Vestibular schwannomas generally grow slowly, but the rate of growth varies among individuals, even those within one family.[7,8] Losses in balance and hearing usually develop insidiously, causing a slow deterioration over a period of years. Less often, hearing loss occurs suddenly or hearing worsens and then improves for a time. These situations are thought to occur because the tumor is compressing blood vessels.[9] If vestibular schwannomas are detected early enough, it is now possible to preserve hearing in some individuals with NF2.

Most people with NF2 develop other types of tumors, yet these seldom become malignant. Because these tumors associated with NF2 originate in the brain and spinal cord, they can result in significant disability and even death. One of these tumors may cause the individual to experience a deterioration or loss of sight, have trouble walking, and be subjected to chronic pain. Some people experience such slow tumor growth that disability is minimal; others experience rapid tumor growth and loss of function. In the most severe cases—fortunately, quite rare—tumors compress the brainstem, causing death.

It is important to note several caveats, however. Because of the strong genotype-phenotype correlation in NF2, the disorder tends to manifest the same way in members of the same family. As a result the general rules may not apply; it is best for patients and physicians to use family history as a guide to what symptoms will develop, and when, in a person with NF2. Improvements in imaging and surgical techniques in the past decade have also enabled clinicians to detect tumors when they are small, sometimes even before they cause symptoms, which in many cases improves outcome.

Some studies have reported that the average life span for someone with NF2 is significantly shorter than for a person in the general population. These conclusions were largely based on old data and may not be relevant now that imaging and surgical techniques have improved. Many people with NF2 live a long time. One often-cited study[3] published in 1992 found that the mean life span in people with NF2 was 62 years—meaning that half died before age 62 and half afterward. Those who died before age 62 tended to die young; the mean age at death for this group in the study was 36. Most early deaths resulted from complications related to NF2.

The same team recently conducted another analysis and probed the issue further.[7] They found that these three clinical factors increased risk of early death: age at diagnosis; where treatment takes place; and presence of meningiomas, a type of brain tumor (see below). The younger a person was at time of diagnosis, the greater the risk of mortality, possibly because earlier age of onset is associated with faster tumor growth. Intracranial meningiomas may pose challenges because they require complicated surgical treatment and proper postoperative care. The authors speculate that patients with NF2 who are treated at specialty clinics are less likely to die because practice and experience are vitally important in surgery. Patients treated at such specialty centers tend to have better treatment outcomes and fewer postoperative complications.

◆ Clinical Features

A brief description of the types of tumors and other manifestations associated with NF2 is provided below. An estimated timetable of when they are most likely to occur is listed in Table **10–2**. Information on management of such manifestations is provided in Chapter 11.

Vestibular Schwannomas

Tumors of the eighth cranial nerve occur in 95% of adults who have NF2 and usually develop on nerves on both sides of the head.[3,5,10] Originally known as acoustic neuromas, these hallmark tumors of NF2 have since been designated "vestibular schwannomas" to reflect a better understanding of their origin and pathology.

Table 10–2   NF2 Features Through the Life Span

Childhood:

Schwannomas visible on skin (subtle)

Eye problems:

- Cataracts (common)
- Congenital amblyopia and strabismus (less common)
- Retinal hamartomas and epiretinal membranes (less common)

Adulthood:

- Bilateral vestibular schwannomas (may develop in late teens; in rare cases, even earlier)
- Spinal and other schwannomas
- Meningiomas
- Ependymomas and astrocytomas

A vestibular schwannoma originates along the vestibular branch of the eighth cranial nerve, which helps people to maintain balance, and therefore may cause symptoms such as dizziness and stumbling. In many cases these initial symptoms escape notice. One exceedingly worrisome and potentially fatal early symptom is that a person who has NF2 may become disoriented while under water (see Chapter 11). As the tumor continues to grow, it places pressure on and sometimes engulfs the other segment of the eighth cranial nerve, the auditory branch. This causes the symptoms that most often prompt people to seek medical attention—ringing in the ears and increasing difficulty with hearing—and explains why these tumors were originally known as acoustic neuromas.

Pathologically the tumors that define NF2 are schwannomas, benign tumors that develop from the Schwann cells that help to form the protective myelin sheath around nerve cells in the central nervous system. Unlike neurofibromas in NF1, which consist of multiple cell types and sometimes infiltrate and become entwined with nerve fibers, schwannomas consist mainly of one cell type and grow within a fibrous capsule that prevents them from growing into the nerve fiber itself. Schwannomas cause symptoms once they grow large enough to compress the nerves and adjacent blood vessels.

Schwannomas Located Elsewhere

Spinal Schwannomas

These tumors are the most common type of spinal tumor seen in NF2, developing in as many as four in five people with the disorder. Most spinal schwannomas are small, do not cause symptoms, and do not require surgery.[11] Spinal schwannomas that develop in the topmost (cervical) and middle (thoracic) portions of the spine may take on a dumbbell shape as they grow, making them indistinguishable in imaging scans from neurofibromas seen in NF1. Multiple small spinal schwannomas may dot the cauda equina, the bundle of nerves located at the lower end of the spinal cord. Although on imaging studies this may resemble metastatic cancer, most spinal schwannomas are benign and do not cause medical complications.

Cranial Schwannomas

One in four people with NF2 will also develop schwannomas on other cranial nerves.[3,5] The fifth cranial (trigeminal) nerve is most often the site. This is the largest cranial nerve, with three branches; it conveys sensory information in the head and face, and one nerve branch helps to control the muscles used in chewing and eating. Tumors on this nerve may grow into the cavernous sinus, a cavity at the base of the skull. Tumors of the third cranial nerve (oculomotor) may cause double vision (diplopia) and lazy eye (amblyopia). When tumors attach to the lower cranial nerves they may cause difficulty in swallowing and cause fluid to enter the lung during an intake of breath *(aspiration)*.

Peripheral Schwannomas

Although NF2 primarily produces tumors in the brain and spinal cord, schwannomas sometimes develop on peripheral nerves that emanate from the spinal cord. Tumors on the major deep nerves in the arms and legs are most likely to cause pain, weakness, and other symptoms. About half of all people with NF2 develop nodular schwannomas in the limbs and trunk that become painful after a minor trauma,[10] such as banging an arm or leg.

Dermal Schwannomas

About half of people with NF2 develop these tumors on the surface of the skin,[3,5,12] although they are usually so subtle that they may be missed. They form as slightly elevated areas of skin, sometimes rough in texture. Skin schwannomas cause no physical effects.

Meningiomas

Meningiomas are tumors that develop in the membrane that covers the surface of the brain and spinal cord. These tumors occur in about half of all people with NF2, more often in the brain than in the spine.[3,5] In most cases, meningiomas are slow growing and may not cause symptoms for years or even decades. When symptoms do occur, they are usually caused by increased pressure within the skull. Pressure results either because the tumor has grown, or because it prevents proper drainage of cerebrospinal fluid from the ventricles, causing fluid to build up in the brain (hydrocephalus). The exact symptoms experienced depend on the tumor's location, but generally they include headaches, nausea, vomiting, and vision complications. Depending on their location, meningiomas may cause changes in mood, personality, speech, coordination, and memory.

Astrocytomas and Ependymomas

Astrocytomas and ependymomas are both tumors that develop from the glial cells that support nerve cells in the brain and spinal cord. Astrocytomas develop from cells known as astrocytes, and usually occur in the brain. Ependymomas develop from ependymal cells that are found in the internal canal of the spinal cord and the ventricles of the brain. Astrocytomas and ependymomas occur less frequently than the other tumors associated with NF2, but it is not known exactly how often they occur. Some studies have estimated that as many as one in three people with NF2 develop such tumors,[11] but only a small percentage of these cause symptoms.

As with any type of brain tumor, symptoms of astrocytomas and ependymomas may include headache, vomiting, and altered vision because of increased pressure inside the skull. Depending on the location of the tumor, there may be changes in mood, personality, speech, writing, coordination, and memory. Symptoms specific to ependymomas include neck pain, optic nerve swelling, and jerky eye movements.

◆ Eye Conditions

Vision complaints are common in people with NF2. Various studies report that some type of visual impairment is a consequence in anywhere from 33 to 75% of people with the disorder.[10,13,14] Because these eye conditions tend to develop before vestibular schwannomas do, they can help establish a diagnosis early on, especially in someone with a family history of NF2.

Cataracts (Fig. **10–1**), cloudy areas that occur in the lens of the eye, are the most frequent ocular complication of NF2. Although cataracts occur in

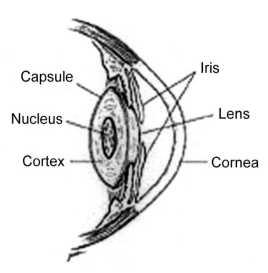

Figure 10–1 A diagram showing where cataracts can form. Nuclear cataract occurs at the lens center (nucleus). Cortical cataract forms in the intermediate cells (cortex) of the lens. And posterior subcapsular cataract (PSC) starts under the outer membrane (capsule) at the back of the lens. (From Harvard Women's Health Watch, May 2002, with permission.)

many people with NF2, they impair vision in only one in five individuals.[6(p306)] When cataracts develop, vision may become cloudy and blurred, and the person may have difficulty dealing with bright lights or glare. Such symptoms develop because the cataract interferes with the focus of light on the retina, the part of the eye that sends visual signals to the brain. The most common types of cataract seen in NF2 are juvenile posterior subcapsular lenticular opacity, a lesion that occurs near the lens cortex and adjacent to the lens capsule, and cortical cataracts, opacities of the lens cortex.

Retinal abnormalities include benign vascular lesions known as hamartomas and the development of a thin film of tissue on the retina known as an epiretinal membrane. About one in four people with NF2 develop retinal abnormalities.[6(p306)] These lesions may sometimes impair vision or cause detachment of the retina.

Strabismus and amblyopia present in one in 10 children with NF2, although it is not clear why. In strabismus, one eye turns in a way that is different from the other when the child looks at something. The eye may turn inward (cross-eye), outward (walleye), or up or down. This type of deviation generally reflects a defect in the brain's ability to keep both eyes aligned and can be corrected. Although babies younger than 6 months may experience occasional strabismus because their eyes have not yet fully developed, the condition is abnormal in older children and should be evaluated.

Amblyopia is sometimes caused by strabismus, but it reflects a different underlying factor: the brain is not able to receive or interpret signals from the eye. This may occur because of defects in nerve connections or because the brain suppresses information coming from an eye misaligned in strabismus. If amblyopia is not detected and treated by the time a child is 2, it is possible that the child will lose sight in the eye and normal depth perception.

Orbital meningiomas are tumors that extend from the brain into the area behind the eye known as the orbit. These tumors may place pressure on the optic nerve, causing vision abnormalities and the eye to bulge outward (proptosis). About 5 to 10% of people with NF2 develop these tumors and need to be monitored to gauge progression.[13,14]

◆ Guidelines for Diagnosis

Diagnosis of NF2 is challenging for several reasons. Most primary care physicians never encounter someone with the disorder; during their career, others may diagnose only one or two cases. Another challenge is that tumors associated with NF2 occur frequently enough in the general population that a physician may not at first suspect NF2 in a person without a family history of the disorder. Noticeably common are vestibular schwannomas that develop on one side of the head. In only 5% of people with unilateral tumors is NF2 eventually diagnosed.[15] Finally, the signs and symptoms of NF2 may be subtle for years. For all these reasons, clinical observations and medical test results must be analyzed in tandem, often for years, to correctly arrive at a diagnosis.

In children with a family history of NF2, the initiation and timing of screening depend on family history; age of onset tends to be the same from one generation to the next. Screening should begin early in children born to families with early-onset NF2, and continue later in life for people born to families with late-onset NF2. In either type of family, initial screening should begin by the time the child reaches puberty. This should include an annual physical and neurological evaluation and an annual magnetic resonance imaging (MRI) scan to detect vestibular schwannomas. In early-onset families, a normal MRI at age 18 indicates that the individual may not develop NF2, and a normal MRI at 30 offers confirmation. In late-onset families, screening should continue even after 30 years of age.[4(p55)]

As discussed in Chapter 4, genetic testing is sometimes useful in early diagnosis of children who have inherited the gene that causes NF2. These tests are not yet accurate enough to be useful in all situations, however. Current tests find the *NF2* mutation in only about six in 10 people who have the disorder. A child with a family history of NF2 who tests negative for the disorder's gene mutation therefore needs to undergo screening until early adulthood. On the other hand, if a genetic test confirms that a child has NF2, anticipatory screening can commence. Screening allows for earlier detection of tumors and presumably better outcomes.

Screening can be more relaxed for individuals with a presumptive diagnosis but no family history of NF2 because their tumors may not be caused by the disorder. These individuals should be evaluated annually for another 5 to 10 years, at which point screening can stop if no further manifestations develop.[4(p54)]

Medical History

When reviewing the medical history of a person suspected of having NF2, the focus is on hallmark symptoms of hearing and coordination difficulties, although other telltale manifestations and overall health should also be discussed. Because there is often a lag between onset of symptoms and diagnosis, it is important to determine when symptoms first began, how they first came to attention, how quickly they progressed, and whether they occurred in tandem with other symptoms (balance abnormalities and hearing difficulties, for instance). If possible, the patient should bring, and the physician review, medical records to document early symptoms and establish a timeline. A thorough medical history for NF2 should include the following topics, which may be revisited in subsequent evaluations:

Hearing

Questions about a patient's hearing should focus on subtle signs of deterioration as well as more obvious indicators of hearing loss. Sometimes the first sign is difficulty in hearing people on the phone when the receiver is placed against one ear or the other. Other early signs may be a constant ringing or roaring in the ears known as tinnitus, or hearing a person speaking at one side of the patient but not at the other.

Balance

Because vestibular schwannomas first develop on the part of the nerve that controls balance, any experience with dizziness, unsteadiness, or difficulties in balance and coordination should be noted. Often these changes are subtle and may be recognized only in hindsight. Some people recall having trouble walking at night over rough terrain, for instance.

Pain

Unexplained persistent pain, and where it occurs, should be noted. Although most tumors in NF2 are located in the central nervous system, pain may be felt elsewhere in the body.

Muscle Weakness

Numbness or weakness should be noted. The face most often sustains the effects of tumors growing on the cranial nerves, but limbs may be jeopardized by spinal tumors.

Vision

Loss or changes in vision should be noted, and referral made to an ophthalmologist for further testing if necessary.

Skin

Unusual bumps or areas of rough skin noticed by the patient should be noted, especially in children with a family history of NF2. Subtle skin schwannomas are an early manifestation of NF2 that often elude detection until other signs develop.

Persistent Headaches and Seizures

Although these symptoms of NF2 occur much less frequently than others, it is helpful to note whether they have occurred. Either may indicate the presence of a brain tumor.

Family Medical History

Because NF2 is inherited in about half of all cases, the medical history of close relatives is relevant when making a diagnosis. One diagnostic criterion is having a first-degree relative with the disorder: a parent, sibling, or child. Because milder forms of NF2 may never have been diagnosed, however, it is important to ask about second-degree relatives: grandparents, aunts, uncles, and cousins, and even their descendants. If NF2 is suspected in any of the patient's first- and second-degree relatives, a diagnosis should be confirmed through medical records and, if possible, physical examination of these relatives.

Physical Examination

Physical evaluation of someone suspected of having NF2 should be done in conjunction with medical tests: physical clues alone are not sufficient to determine diagnosis. This is especially true in someone with no family history of the disorder.

Skin Features

Although more subtle than the dermatological manifestations of NF1, certain skin features are associated with NF2. Skin schwannomas (Fig. **10–2**)

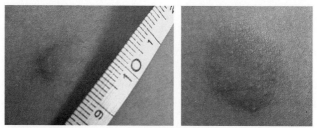

Figure 10–2   A skin schwannoma seen in a child with NF2. (From Nunes F, MacCollin M. Neurofibromatosis 2 in the pediatric population. J Child Neurol 2003;18:718–724, with permission.)

may appear as small bumps or areas of roughened skin anywhere on the body, including the scalp. Hair sprouting from a schwannoma may be darker and coarser than surrounding hair. Skin schwannomas develop early in childhood and, unlike neurofibromas in NF1, do not become significantly larger or more numerous with time.

Multiple café-au-lait spots may be visible, and perhaps larger and more numerous than in the general population, but they are not so distinctive that they can be used in diagnosis. People with NF2 do not have the six or more café-au-lait spots indicative of NF1.

Neurological Evaluation

Neurological assessment should focus on vestibular function by testing balance and coordination, and provide an assessment of cranial nerve and spinal cord function. Many people with NF2 exhibit areflexia, a condition in which reflexes are muted or absent. In rare cases, people with NF2 may also develop peripheral neuropathy, a loss of sensation in the extremities, and mononeuritis multiplex, a dysfunction of isolated nerves in several areas of the body.

Ophthalmological Evaluation

Anyone diagnosed with, or suspected of having, NF2 should have a thorough eye examination annually. This should include predominant attention to the iris and the lens, because that is where cataracts and other abnormalities described earlier develop (Fig. **10–3**). People with NF2 do not develop Lisch nodules, which are associated with NF1. However, if there is any doubt about the diagnosis, a slit-lamp examination to detect such lesions should be included in the evaluation. It is also important to test vision and assess the health of the optic nerve, to detect the presence of tumors. These are most often orbital meningiomas; the optic gliomas seen in NF1 do not occur in people with NF2.

Additional Testing

Medical tests to supplement physical examination are essential for diagnosis and management of NF2.

Audiogram

An *audiogram* is a graph that charts the results of hearing tests to show how well a person hears (Fig. **10–4**). Low- to high-pitch sounds are charted horizontally from left to right, whereas soft to loud sounds are charted vertically from top to bottom. Hearing is then measured in

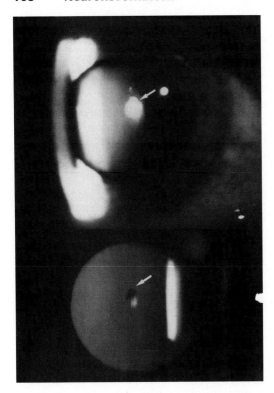

Figure 10–3   Posterior subcapsular cataract (arrow) in patient with NF2 seen on dilated biomicroscopy of the right lens. (Courtesy of Muriel I. Kaiser-Kupfer, M.D., National Eye Institute, National Institutes of Health, with permission.)

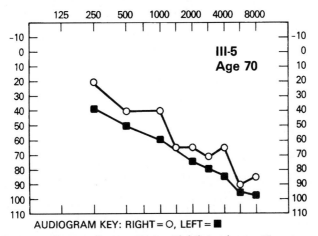

Figure 10–4   Audiogram from patient with bilateral acoustic neuromas, showing 20- to 40-dB sensorineural hearing loss at 250 Hz, increasing to 80 to 100 dB at 8000 Hz. The left side is worse than the right. (Courtesy of Anita T. Pikus, Au.D., president of Zebra System International [ZSI], based on data obtained while she was chief of clinical audiology at the National Institute on Deafness and Other Communication Disorders, National Institutes of Health, with permission.)

decibels, and a threshold is established to determine the softest sounds the patient can hear. Thresholds of 0 to 20 or 25 dB are considered normal; anything over that range may indicate hearing loss. The higher a person's threshold, the more extensive is hearing loss. A thorough audiological assessment should include pure tone audiometry. Many people with NF2 experience high-frequency hearing loss. Additional tests gauge the ability to hear spoken words and discriminate among different tones.

Brainstem Auditory Evoked Response (BAER)

A BAER records the electrical activity generated in the brain in response to selected sounds and is used to assess the health of the auditory nerve (Fig. **10–5**). This test is highly sensitive and may therefore provide an early indication of hearing loss, long before the person notices any changes. The person being tested wears earphones that emit clicking noises or tones, while electrical activity is monitored through electrodes placed on the scalp.

Cranial Magnetic Resonance Imaging

If audiometry tests and BAER indicate any hearing loss in a person suspected of having NF2, a cranial MRI (Fig. **10–6**) helps to determine the

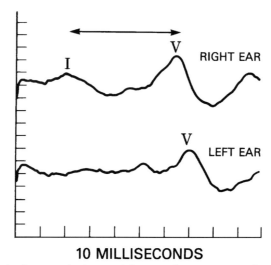

10 MILLISECONDS

Figure 10–5   Auditory evoked potential tracing from patient with NF2. Right wave I to V interpeak interval of 4.47 msec is more than 2.5 standard deviations beyond the clinical norm of 3.95 msec. Left I to V interpeak interval could not be measured. (Courtesy of Anita T. Pikus, Au.D., president of Zebra System International [ZSI], based on data obtained while she was chief of clinical audiology at the National Institute on Deafness and Other Communication Disorders, National Institutes of Health, with permission.)

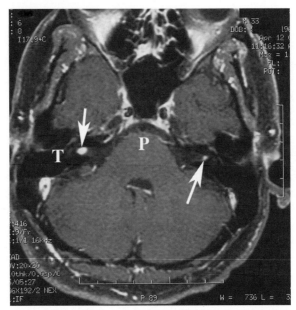

Figure 10–6   Bilateral vestibular schwannomas (BVSs) are the hallmark of NF2 and originate within the temporal bones (T) on the eighth cranial nerve. If left untreated, these small asymptomatic tumors (arrows) will grow inward and compress the brainstem at the level of the pons (P). (Courtesy of Mia MacCollin, M.D., Massachusetts General Hospital, with permission.)

cause. MRI remains the gold standard in detecting these tumors, even when they are too small to cause symptoms. To ensure that a vestibular schwannoma is accurately detected, the following parameters are necessary during the MRI[4(p54)]:

- Image slices should be taken at 3-mm intervals through the internal auditory canals. This helps to detect even small tumors.
- Images should be taken both with and without gadolinium, a tracer that helps to enhance the image.
- It is important to take both axial (a view from the top of the skull) and coronal (a view from the front of the skull) images with fat saturation (a technical term for one of several radiofrequency pulses used to create MRI images).

Spinal Magnetic Resonance Imaging

Full spinal MRI images, with and without gadolinium enhancement, should be taken in anyone newly diagnosed with NF2. If ependymomas or astrocytomas are detected, annual follow-up spinal MRIs are recommended, unless the development of symptoms indicates the need for

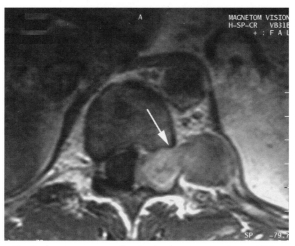

Figure 10–7   Typical appearance of spinal schwannoma in an NF2 patient. The tumor has originated within the neuroforamen (arrow) and has assumed a "dumbbell" configuration with tumor mass both in and out of the spinal canal itself. T1-weighted, contrast enhanced axial MRI scan. (Courtesy of Mia MacCollin, M.D., Massachusetts General Hospital, with permission.)

more frequent scans. If spinal schwannomas and spinal meningiomas are detected on an initial MRI (Fig. **10–7**), follow-up screening images are not necessary unless a person with NF2 experiences pain, numbness, or other symptoms that would suggest the tumor is pressing on nerves. Even when these tumors do cause ramifications, symptoms usually worsen gradually. If any new tumors appear, follow-up should take place every 6 to 12 months to monitor growth.[4(pp54,55)]

Spinal MRIs are also appropriate in someone suspected of having NF2, especially if there is unexplained numbness or weakness that might be caused by a spinal tumor. The detection of NF2-related tumors in the spine, even if they do not cause symptoms, can help to confirm a diagnosis.

Biopsy

A preliminary operation to remove only a portion of a tumor (a biopsy) is done only in the case of peripheral tumors. If surgery is required for brain and spinal cord tumors, the entire mass will be removed during an operation.

Genetic Testing

Clinical testing is sometimes helpful in confirming a diagnosis. Such testing is available only when requested by a physician and at a limited number of sites.

◆ Differential Diagnosis: Distinguishing Neurofibromatosis 2 from Other Conditions

Differential diagnosis is a process that a physician goes through when there is any doubt about diagnosis. Conditions similar to NF2 are considered, their manifestations reviewed, and then a determination is made about whether a person's manifestations more closely resemble NF2 or these other disorders. The most common conditions that are similar to NF2 are briefly reviewed below.

Segmental or Mosaic NF2

As is the case with NF1, sometimes the gene that causes NF2 mutates after the zygote forms at conception. Only those tissues that develop from the mutated cell express the NF2 characteristics. As a result, the individual may develop features of NF2, but only in one part of the body.

People who develop unilateral vestibular schwannomas may have mosaic NF2, especially if any additional NF2-related tumors develop only on one side of the body. Some studies suggest that even people with bilateral vestibular schwannomas may have mosaic NF2 if the tumors on one side of the head are much bigger or smaller than those on the other side. It is also possible that extremely mild cases of NF2 may in fact be the result of postzygotic mutations.

There is no way of knowing whether the eggs or sperm of someone with segmental NF2 harbor the causative gene mutation. For that reason, people with the mosaic form of the disorder risk passing the generalized form of NF2 on to children.

Unilateral Vestibular Schwannoma

If there is no family history of NF2, a schwannoma revealed on the vestibular nerve on just one side of the head may represent a sporadic tumor—one that develops by chance. Ninety-five percent of unilateral vestibular schwannomas are in fact sporadic tumors,[9] and these are surprisingly common, accounting for 5 to 10%[16] of all brain tumors in the general population. In addition to family history, age of onset can help a physician to assess whether a unilateral vestibular schwannoma may be a sign of NF2. If such a tumor is found in someone younger than 25, careful screening is advised. If it develops in someone older than 55, NF2 is most likely not related to it.[9]

Multiple Meningiomas

Sometimes two or more meningiomas develop in people without NF2, either by chance or because they inherited a rare familial syndrome that is caused by a gene other than the one responsible for NF2. Age of onset can help a physician to determine whether the meningiomas may be associated with NF2 or unrelated to the disorder. Because sporadic meningiomas most often occur in older adults, anyone who develops such a tumor before age 25 should have an NF2 evaluation.[9] In NF2, meningiomas rarely develop before vestibular schwannomas. If an MRI of the eighth cranial nerve finds no vestibular schwannomas, it is likely that the person does not have NF2.

Schwannomatosis

As discussed in Chapter 12, this disorder is genetically distinct from NF2 but is often confused with it. People with schwannomatosis develop multiple schwannomas on nerves everywhere except on the eighth cranial nerve. These tumors may develop in the spine and in the peripheral nerves. If someone presents with them, a first step in determining whether it is NF2 or schwannomatosis is to conduct an MRI of the eighth cranial nerve, to determine whether it also has a schwannoma. Questions about symptoms further help to distinguish the two disorders. People with NF2 tend to experience more pronounced neurological deficits, such as hearing loss and impaired coordination, but are less likely to experience pain, whereas people with schwannomatosis tend to experience more pronounced pain and less neurological disability.

◆ The Personal Perspective

Adam G.: "I was 10 years old when I was diagnosed with NF2. I am the first one in my family to have this disorder. There were early signs, but they were missed. I had tinnitus, a ringing in my ears, already by that time. When we look back at pictures of me, my left eye always was pushed out a little. Nobody ever noticed. The biggest symptom I had was that I was 25% deaf in my left ear, but no one realized the significance. The hearing loss had been noted, but no one put it together.

"I don't remember which doctor diagnosed it. I was originally misdiagnosed with tuberous sclerosis [a genetic disorder that is evident in the skin and nervous system and sometimes causes tumor growth]. I was going for an eye checkup. Because they thought I had tuberous sclerosis, they were doing extra tests and discovered a growth behind my left eye. Then they did more MRI scans. It turns out that they missed the tumors earlier because the MRI slices they'd taken were too wide. At that time the tumors were small. So then they properly diagnosed it as NF2."

Martha L.: "I was 19 years old and started to notice that with my right ear I was having difficulty understanding people on the phone. My parents took me to see two different neurologists/neurosurgeons to find out what was happening to me. This was in 1987, when NF2 was not very well known. These two doctors didn't have a clue as to what was wrong with me. They dropped us like hot potatoes, to avoid their own embarrassment at not being able to figure out why this was occurring. They never made themselves available to us, never returned my parents' phone calls, or anything.

"My father, who is a radiologist, spoke with his college roommate who is a neurosurgeon in California. He knew what it was when my dad told him about my symptoms. He suggested we go out and see him. He said it would be easier on my parents if he told me personally what was wrong, and why. We flew out to see him and, on a separate meeting, met with another ear and hearing specialist.

"It was a neurosurgeon in Boston who really made an impact on me. The initial visit was probably almost a year after I started to notice a change in my hearing. That's how much time we wasted on those other ignorant doctors. My hearing started to get much worse, very quickly. I would get so angry. Maybe frustrated and scared is a better description about what was happening to me. My neurosurgeon would be so kind and gentle in trying to explain things, but I would get mad and just storm out of his office because I couldn't deal with the hearing loss. He stuck right by me no matter what, with that same gentle manner of his, and he knew it wasn't personal. It was then that I started to realize how much I could trust him. He was going to be there no matter what, and not avoid us like those other doctors. To this day, I consider him my hero, because he was there to explain this whole frightening thing, was always available to us, and performed major surgeries on me, which I always came out of successfully."

References

1. National Institutes of Health. NIH. Neurofibromatosis Consensus Conference. Neurofibromatosis Conference Statement. Arch Neurol 1988;45:575–578
2. National Institutes of Health Conference. Neurofibromatosis 1 (Recklinghausen disease) and neurofibromatosis 2 (bilateral acoustic neurofibromatosis): an update. Ann Intern Med 1990;113:39–52
3. Evans DG, Huson SM, Donnai D, et al. A clinical study of type 2 neurofibromatosis. Q J Med 1992;84:603–618
4. Gutmann DH, Aylsworth A, Carey JC, et al. The diagnostic evaluation and multidisciplinary management of

neurofibromatosis 1 and neurofibromatosis 2. JAMA 1997;278:51–57

5. Parry DM, Eldridge R, Kaiser-Kupfer MI, Bouzas EA, Pikus A, Patronas N. Neurofibromatosis 2 (NF2): clinical characteristics of 63 affected individuals and clinical evidence for heterogeneity. Am J Med Genet 1994;52:450–461

6. Friedman JM, Gutmann DH, MacCollin M, Riccardi VM, eds. Neurofibromatosis: Phenotype, Natural History, and Pathogenesis. 3rd ed. Baltimore: Johns Hopkins University Press; 1999

7. Baser ME, Friedman JM, Aeschliman D, et al. Predictors of the risk of mortality in neurofibromatosis 2. Am J Hum Genet 2002;71:715–723

8. Mautner VF, Baser ME, Thakkar SD, Feigen UM, Friedman JM, Kluwe L. Vestibular schwannoma growth in patients with neurofibromatosis type 2: a longitudinal study. J Neurosurg 2002;96:223–228

9. MacCollin MM. Neurofibromatosis 2. Gene reviews [serial online]. October 29, 2001. Available at: http://www.geneclinics.org.

10. Mautner VF, Lindenau M, Baser M, et al. The neuroimaging and clinical spectrum of neurofibromatosis 2. Neurosurgery 1996;38:880–886

11. Mautner VF, Tatagiba M, Lindenau M, et al. Spinal tumors in patients with neurofibromatosis type 2: MR imaging study of frequency, multiplicity, and variety. AJR Am J Roentgenol 1995;165:951–955

12. Mautner VF, Lindenau M, Baser ME, Kluwe L, Gottschalk J. Skin abnormalities in neurofibromatosis 2. Arch Dermatol 1997;133:1539–1543

13. Bouzas EA, Parry DM, Eldridge R, Kaiser-Kupfer MI. Visual impairment in patients with neurofibromatosis 2. Neurology 1993;43:622–623

14. Ragge NK, Baser ME, Klein J, et al. Ocular abnormalities in neurofibromatosis 2. Am J Ophthalmol 1995;120:634–641

15. Eldridge R, Parry D. Vestibular schwannoma (acoustic neuroma). Consensus development conference. Neurosurgery 1992;30:962–964

16. Bruce J, Fetell M. Tumors of the skull and cranial nerves. In: Rowland LP, ed. Merritt's Textbook of Neurology. 9th ed. Baltimore: Williams & Wilkins; 1995:320. Cited in MacCollin MM. Neurofibromatosis 2. Gene reviews [serial online]. October 29, 2001. Available at: http://www.geneclinics.org.

11

Management of Particular Neurofibromatosis 2 Features

A diagnosis of confirmed or probable neurofibromatosis 2 (NF2) raises a host of new challenges. Optimal management of the disorder depends on several variables, including the individual's age, family history, symptoms, and comfort with risk. Problems with vision are best treated early, but that is not always the case with tumors. Because the tumors associated with NF2 are usually slow growing, treatment decisions are complicated. The patient and physicians together must weigh the risks and benefits of treatment carefully, including the timing of intervention and the type of surgery chosen. The risk/benefit ratio also depends on the type of tumor being discussed. Early intervention might be proposed in treating vestibular schwannomas, for instance, to increase the chances of hearing preservation. A strategy of watchful waiting might be more appropriate for other sorts of brain and spinal tumors associated with NF2.

In general, optimal management in NF2 should take place at a specialty clinic and consists of anticipatory screening for people with confirmed or probable diagnoses who remain asymptomatic. Such screening may occur more frequently when a person is first diagnosed, to determine how quickly tumors are growing. In most people annual follow-up evaluations are sufficient, following the guidelines in Chapter 10. This chapter reviews the issues and options that arise when manifestations develop.

◆ Vestibular Schwannomas

The hallmark tumors of NF2, vestibular schwannomas, eventually require treatment in most cases. The decision about whether to perform surgery depends on several factors such as the age of the person and the rate at which the tumors are growing. Vestibular schwannomas can eventually grow so large that they engulf the eighth cranial nerve, resulting in hearing loss and other complications. They can also damage other cranial nerves and cause facial paralysis, brainstem compression, and ultimately even death.

A key challenge is to decide how early to intervene and what technique to use. In the past, concern about the risks of surgery—which could itself cause hearing loss—convinced many surgeons that the best strategy was to wait until the tumors grew large enough to cause significant hearing impairment before removing them. With the advent of improved imaging and surgical techniques, opinion on this matter is changing. Many experts now recommend a more proactive approach, with intervention initiated early in an attempt to preserve hearing. It is important to note, however, that the issue remains controversial and the exact strategy chosen involves an individual assessment of risks and benefits for each individual case.

Management options for vestibular schwannomas now fall into three broad categories: surgical removal, radiation, and monitoring.

Surgery

There are several surgical options, depending on tumor size and extent of hearing loss. Some techniques preserve the auditory nerve and enable the patient to retain some hearing; others may sacrifice the nerve but are combined with insertion of an electronic auditory brainstem implant to restore hearing.

In general, people with small vestibular schwannomas (defined as less than 1.5 cm) that are contained within the internal auditory canal are likely to retain hearing following total surgical removal of the tumor.[1,2] Recommendations vary about how to treat people with larger tumors who still retain some functional hearing. Some experts recommend partial tumor removal to preserve hearing,[3] whereas others think that total tumor removal is appropriate for people with tumors less than 2.5 cm in diameter, as long as it is done in a way to preserve hearing.[4] (The surgical options are explained below.)

If a person has bilateral tumors and still has functional hearing, one tumor may be treated first and the results assessed 6 to 12 months later. This allows time to see whether hearing was preserved in the treated ear before intervention decisions are made about the remaining ear. If hearing has been lost in the treated ear, patient and physician may decide on a strategy of watchful waiting to preserve hearing in the remaining ear for as long as possible.[5]

Total tumor removal is accomplished by several techniques. People who have sustained significant hearing loss may undergo translabyrinthine craniotomy. This procedure removes the auditory nerve along with the tumor, causing complete deafness in the ear. In some people, hearing may be partially restored by implanting an auditory brainstem implant. The suboccipital approach is generally used for people whose tumors have not yet extended into the internal auditory canal. The middle cranial fossa method may be best for people with small tumors and functional hearing; it results in hearing preservation in a significant number of people.[4]

Partial tumor removal, also known as decompression, may be an option for people whose tumors are being monitored and who are experiencing fluctuations in hearing. The usual technique is the middle fossa approach, which involves the removal of some bone and tissue so that the tumor can continue to grow without compressing the cochlear and auditory nerves. This restores hearing in some people, at least temporarily. Generally this procedure is not recommended, however, because eventually another operation must be done to remove the tumor, and long-term risk of hearing loss is about the same as in total tumor removal.[4]

Although surgical techniques have improved significantly in recent years, risks remain. Sometimes facial nerves are damaged during surgery, causing temporary or permanent numbness and drooping (palsy) on one side of the face. This can cause additional consequences, such as corneal damage due to an inability to blink, or trouble chewing food. Some people also experience temporary or chronic headaches following brain surgery.

Radiation

Radiation therapy has also improved with the advent of stereotactic devices, such as the gamma knife, that enable radiosurgeons to precisely target the tumor while sparing surrounding healthy tissue. In radiation therapy, high-energy x-rays damage genetic material in cells so that they can no longer divide and multiply. These damaged cells eventually die. Stereotactic radiosurgery is based on the same principle, but enables multiple beams to converge on the tumor from different angles. This increases total dose delivered to the tumor while minimizing the amount that spills over into surrounding tissue.

Radiation therapy does not completely destroy the tumor, but it may shrink it and prevent or retard further growth. This allows hearing preservation in many people. Although sometimes viewed as a "miracle" treatment, radiotherapy is not appropriate for every patient. In some circumstances, radiotherapy may provide an additional treatment option, especially for people who do not want to undergo conventional surgery or are not eligible for it because of age, medical history, or some other reason. A risk to consider is that any radiation treatment may initiate a malignant transformation in the treated tumor.

Monitoring

Once the mainstay of management for vestibular schwannomas, a strategy of watchful waiting is now reserved only for selected individuals with NF2. These include people who are unlikely to benefit from attempts at hearing preservation, individuals who have already lost hearing in one ear, and patients who are too old or ill to tolerate surgery. The person in question should undergo a magnetic resonance imaging (MRI) scan annually to monitor growth and progression of the tumor. Surgery is initiated once hearing is lost or the tumor becomes so large that it threatens further disability.

Counseling

The person who sustains significant or total hearing loss may be devastated. Given the risks that some degree of hearing loss may occur in NF2, even after vestibular schwannomas are treated, it is wise to discuss what options are available besides an auditory brainstem implant. Lip reading and sign language are two longstanding alternatives. Both techniques are easier to learn while some functional hearing remains. Any patient who is experiencing hearing loss and/or considering treatment of vestibular schwannomas should ask for a consultation with an audiologist to review all the options and decide whether to begin training in lip reading or sign language.

Although loss of hearing is often a primary concern for people with NF2, anyone with vestibular schwannomas should also receive counseling about the potential challenges posed by loss of vestibular nerve function. This includes dizziness, unsteadiness while walking, and disorientation while under water. The last point is exceptionally important; some people with bilateral vestibular schwannomas have drowned while swimming.[6] People with NF2 should not take up diving and should swim only when accompanied by others.

◆ Hearing Implants in Neurofibromatosis 2

Some surgical techniques to remove vestibular schwannomas sever the auditory nerve. When this occurs, an electronic device known as an auditory brainstem implant may restore partial hearing in some people. Conventional hearing aids and cochlear implants are not effective.

To understand why, it is first necessary to understand how people hear (Fig. **11–1**). Sound travels into the outer ear to the eardrum, which vibrates in response. Three small bones in the middle ear known as ossicles (the anvil, hammer, and stirrup) start to move as a result, and they convert sound waves into mechanical pressure that is then conveyed to the fluid-filled cochlea. As the fluid begins to move, tiny hairs in the cochlea send electrical signals to the brain via the auditory nerve.

Conventional hearing aids amplify sounds sent to the eardrum. These may be useful early on, when vestibular schwannomas cause limited hearing loss, but will not be helpful over the long term. Cochlear implants bypass damage in this part of the inner ear and directly stimulate the auditory

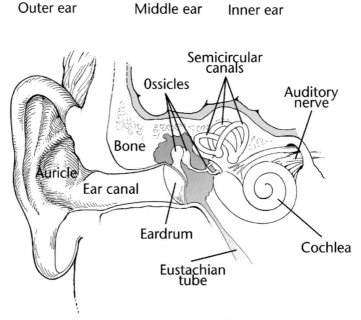

Figure 11–1   Sound travels from the eardrum, where it causes vibrations that are transmitted by the ossicles, into the inner ear. The cochlea transmits sound impulses to the auditory nerve leading to the brain. (Courtesy of Harriet Greenfield, with permission.)

nerve. Neither is effective if the auditory nerve itself is damaged or severed. The auditory brainstem implant is an electronic device implanted on the surface of the cochlear nucleus in the brainstem, thereby bypassing the inner ear. Instead, sounds are sent from the brainstem to the brain.

◆ Treatment of Other Tumors

The other types of schwannomas and tumors that occur in NF2 should be treated only when the symptoms they cause are severe enough to warrant the risk of surgery or radiation therapy. This is because in some instances more disability will result from surgery than from the tumor itself, and radiation therapy carries the risk of malignant transformation.

Other Schwannomas

Cranial Nerve Schwannomas

Schwannomas on other cranial nerves (Fig. **11–2**) are generally treated only when they cause symptoms such as headache and functional deficits,

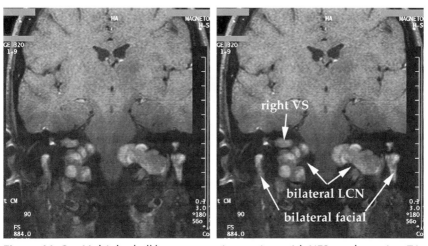

Figure 11–2   Multiple skull base tumors in a patient with NF2, as shown in a T1-weighted, contrast-enhanced, coronal magnetic resonance imaging (MRI) scan. The radiographic appearance of these tumors suggests schwannomas that are growing on the vestibular nerve (VS), the facial nerves, and the lower cranial nerves (LCNs). Skull base tumors may also be meningiomas, or may be abutting meningiomas and schwannomas ("collision" tumors). (Courtesy of Mia MacCollin, M.D., Massachusetts General Hospital, with permission.)

or when they threaten to compress the brainstem. Surgery remains the mainstay of treatment, although radiation therapy may be appropriate for those tumors that cannot be removed surgically.

Spinal Schwannomas

Surgery remains the mainstay of treatment for spinal schwannomas. Options include complete surgical resection or debulking to relieve pressure. Because surgery itself may cause permanent disability or impairment, treatment is recommended only for people experiencing extreme pain or other symptoms.

Peripheral Schwannomas

Schwannomas located on major nerves in the arms and legs are most likely to become painful or cause weakness in the limb. Because schwannomas do not invade the nerve, it is possible to remove many of these tumors without causing significant nerve damage.

Skin Schwannomas

Unlike the dermal tumors seen in NF1, skin schwannomas associated with NF2 do not become larger or more numerous over time. There is no medical reason to remove these tumors, although some people seek treatment for cosmetic reasons.

Astrocytomas and Ependymomas

Some astrocytomas and ependymomas that occur in the general population are treated aggressively with some combination of surgery, radiation, and chemotherapy, especially if they are considered fast growing. When these tumors occur in people with NF2, an aggressive treatment approach is usually not necessary. As do other tumors associated with the disorder, both ependymomas and astrocytomas in NF2 tend to grow slowly and may not cause medical concerns for years. Even then symptoms develop slowly.

Meningiomas

Most meningiomas in people with NF2 (Fig. **11–3**) grow slowly and do not cause symptoms for years. Treatment is recommended when symptoms such as pain and neurological impairment occur, when swelling (edema) develops around the tumor, and when the tumor grows rapidly. Of significant consequence is rapid growth in a tumor near the brainstem, which

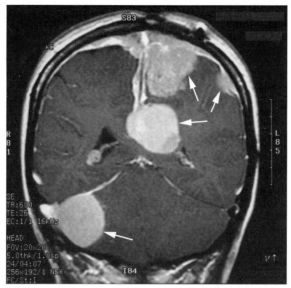

Figure 11–3   Multiple meningiomas in a patient with NF2, as shown in a T1-weighted, contrast-enhanced, coronal MRI scan. Meningiomas are tumors growing from the linings of the brain and in some older NF2 patients can coat nearly every surface in the brain (arrows). (Courtesy of Mia MacCollin, M.D., Massachusetts General Hospital, with permission.)

can cause fluid to build up in the brain (hydrocephalus), and near the eyes, because it can compress the optic nerve and compromise vision.

Treatment depends on the size and location of the tumor, as well as the symptoms. If edema has occurred, steroid drugs may be prescribed to reduce swelling. If the tumor is accessible, surgery is usually the treatment of choice. Radiation therapy may be offered in conjunction with surgery, or used on its own if the tumor cannot be surgically removed.

◆ Management of Eye Conditions in Neurofibromatosis 2

Although much of the focus in NF2 is on management of tumors and preservation of hearing, the disorder also causes ocular manifestations that may require treatment to prevent vision loss. The potentially most damaging of all is an orbital meningioma, which can injure the optic nerve and cause blindness unless detected and treated early.

Cataracts

Most cataracts associated with NF2 do not interfere with vision, but those that do can be managed in one of several ways. When changes such as blurred vision or poor night vision develop, the first strategies may be as simple as a new eyeglass prescription, magnifying lenses, or supplemental lighting. When vision deteriorates to the extent that it interferes with everyday activities such as reading, driving, and working, surgery may be necessary.

Cataract surgery is relatively safe and produces improved vision in most people. Usually this procedure is done on an outpatient basis and involves removal of the clouded lens followed by replacement with an artificial lens. It may take several months for the eye to completely heal. In some cases, a patient is provided with special cataract eyeglasses or a contact lens instead of the replacement lens.

Retinal Abnormalities

Although retinal hamartomas and epiretinal membranes may sometimes progress to the point that they cause losses in vision, in most cases treatment is not necessary. In rare situations, vision may deteriorate to the point to justify vitrectomy, a surgical procedure to remove the lesion or membrane.

Strabismus and Amblyopia

As in the general population, strabismus that develops in someone with NF2 should be treated during childhood to ensure that the eyes make the proper connections with visual pathways in the brain. Strategies include patching the stronger eye to force the weaker one to develop, and use of eyeglasses with special lenses to help the weak eye to better focus. If these strategies do not work, surgery may be necessary. Therapy is similar for amblyopia, but it is most successful when it occurs between ages 6 months and 2 years. This enables the child to make the proper neural connections from the eye to the brain. Therapy may still be effective in providing normal vision for children until age 6; older children show less benefit from intervention.

Orbital Meningiomas

Treatment of orbital meningiomas is usually considered when the tumors cause proptosis, restrict vision, or grow aggressively. In some cases it may be possible to remove the tumor without damaging the optic nerve, but most often the nerve must be sacrificed, causing blindness in the eye.

Sometimes the eye itself must be removed. Radiation therapy is reserved for tumors that cannot be removed surgically.

◆ The Personal Perspective

Adam G: "In 1995, I went to an ear institute to have the tumor on my left auditory nerve removed. They said the odds were that my hearing would be preserved, but I lost my hearing in the left ear. I still have hearing in my right ear. They kept running all sorts of tests and discovered other growths along my spinal cord and on my brainstem. All of the tumors are benign and most are small. Most are inoperable. We might be able to treat them with radiation, but I don't want to go down that road right now.

"They also found a tumor on my left optic nerve. I started losing my peripheral vision and then it progressed so that I had almost no vision. When they took the tumor out, I lost vision completely in that eye. I've had bad luck with surgery.

"I've also got a tumor on my right auditory nerve. Our biggest hope is for an auditory brainstem implant, although I don't know if it will work. They're afraid the nerve might have been injured. At this point, we're just monitoring things."

Martha L.: "My first major surgery was in 1989. My neurosurgeon wanted to try to keep what hearing I had in my left ear by performing decompression surgery. He took out part of the bones in my ear canal so that the tumor would have room to grow and not cause any more harm to my hearing. I was in the hospital for about a week. I couldn't get out of bed for at least a day or two because my balance had been so badly affected. Because he had to cut open my skull, I was placed on an antiseizure medication along with steroids to keep the swelling down. The operation probably prolonged my hearing, but in the end, it didn't really help. The tumor grew in size by only a small amount, but it wound itself so tightly around my ear nerves that it ended up doing harm that way.

"Then in 1994 one of the tumors in my brain was growing and causing really bad headaches. This surgery was the most serious of all. I was convinced I would end up with some paralysis, memory loss, who knows what. My neurosurgeon reassured me as much as possible that I would be fine, and he was right. I woke up knowing who my husband and my parents were, I could feel my arms and legs, and I definitely knew who my neurosurgeon was. He was the one who made everything all better and safe again.

"In 1997 I had a tumor removed from my lower spine. It was causing really bad cramps in my calves, along with lower back pain and weakness.

I don't recall much about what was involved, just that it was pretty simple, in comparison to the other surgery.

"In 1998 my right vestibular schwannoma was growing and I needed surgery. My neurosurgeon said he could perform another major invasive surgery, but that there was a somewhat newer procedure that was noninvasive, had less risk of infection, and required barely any recovery time. It was called gamma knife radiosurgery. The procedure itself was long, but very easy. The worst part about it was having this metal halo screwed into my head so that the radiation would go to the right places. We stayed overnight in a hotel and went home the next day. A follow-up MRI showed the procedure was a success. The tumor was shrinking and not growing any more.

"In 2001 my left vestibular schwannoma and one of the tumors in my brain had both increased in size and needed surgery. The procedure and recovery time were the same during this second gamma knife experience. I think from now on, if I need more surgical intervention, and if it is possible, I will always undergo gamma knife radiosurgery. It is so much easier than invasive surgery. Not only is it quicker, with less recovery time for me, it is a lot less emotional and stressful for my husband and family."

References

1. Briggs RJ, Brackmann DE, Baser ME, Hitselberger WE. Comprehensive management of bilateral acoustic neuromas. Arch Otolaryngol Head Neck Surg 1994;120:1307–1314
2. Ojemann RG. Management of acoustic neuromas (vestibular schwannomas). Clin Neurosurg 1993;40:498–535
3. Gutmann DH, Aylsworth A, Carey JC, et al. The diagnostic evaluation and multidisciplinary management of neurofibromatosis 1 and neurofibromatosis 2. JAMA 1997;278:51–57
4. Brackmann DE, Fayad JN, Slattery WH III, et al. Early proactive management of vestibular schwannomas in neurofibromatosis type 2. Neurosurgery 2001;49:274–280
5. Slattery WH III, Brackmann DE, Hitselberger W. Hearing preservation in neurofibromatosis type 2. Am J Otolaryngol 1998;19:638–643
6. Kanter WR, Eldridge R, Fabricant R, Allen JC, Koerber T. Central neurofibromatosis with bilateral acoustic neuroma: genetic, clinical and biochemical distinctions from peripheral neurofibromatosis. Neurology 1980; 30:851–859

12

Schwannomatosis

Schwannomatosis is a newly recognized form of neurofibromatosis that is distinct from neurofibromatosis 1 (NF1) and neurofibromatosis 2 (NF2), in terms of both its primary clinical features and its genetic basis. As this book went to press, it was not yet clear what gene or mechanism might be responsible for schwannomatosis. For that reason, many basic questions about schwannomatosis remain unanswered. Research into schwannomatosis is yielding new insights every year, however. To obtain the most current information, contact the NF Foundation or visit its Web site: www.nf.org.

People with schwannomatosis develop multiple schwannomas, benign tumors of the myelin sheath that surrounds nerves, anywhere in the body except on the vestibular nerve—the chief clinical feature that differentiates it from NF2. Pain, often excruciating and sometimes disabling in intensity, is the primary symptom experienced by people with schwannomatosis and most often prompts them to seek medical help.

Schwannomatosis was once considered to be so rare that it was described mainly on the basis of "case reports," clinical descriptions of individual patients and isolated families reported in research publications. First described in Japanese patients,[1] schwannomatosis was subsequently diagnosed in other ethnic groups around the world. Although the condition has sometimes been called "neurilemomatosis," the accepted term today is schwannomatosis. Studies indicate that schwannomatosis is as common as NF2, although rare.[2,3]

Although some researchers once argued[4] that schwannomatosis is a variant form of NF2, the consensus now is that it is a distinct type of neurofibromatosis. However, because NF2 and schwannomatosis share a key clinical feature—multiple schwannoma growth—some patients have to be followed for years until a diagnosis can be confirmed.[4-6] To further complicate matters, spinal neurofibromas associated with NF1 appear so similar to spinal schwannomas on imaging tests that the two tumor types can be distinguished only by analyzing excised tissue under a microscope. Case reports indicate that some patients with spinal tumors are inadvertently diagnosed as having NF1, when later tissue analysis indicates that they have schwannomatosis.

◆ Theories of Pathogenesis

It is not yet clear what causes schwannomatosis. Part of the challenge in finding the responsible mechanism is that the inherited or familial version of schwannomatosis accounts for only ~15% of cases; the remainder are sporadic cases that develop without a family history of the disorder.[3] This makes the hunt for the responsible gene or genes more difficult, simply because there are proportionally fewer family pedigrees and blood samples to analyze than there are for NF1 and NF2, which are inherited 50% of the time.

The hunt for the mechanism responsible for schwannomatosis has also been hindered by puzzling and contradictory findings when tumor samples were analyzed in the laboratory. For instance, both copies of the *NF2* gene are inactivated in tumors taken from people with schwannomatosis, suggesting that the same mechanism seen in NF1 and NF2—a loss of a tumor suppressor gene—might be at work.[7] As discussed in Chapter 3, when one copy of a tumor-suppressor gene is malfunctioning in all cells of the body, as it is in NF1 and NF2, then tumor formation begins after the remaining copy of a gene is lost in particular tissues. Based on analysis of tumor samples, some speculated that schwannomatosis might be caused by such a two-hit loss of the *NF2* gene.[4] Researchers have discovered, however, that both copies of the *NF2* gene remain functional in healthy tissue from people with schwannomatosis, which rules out this theory.[8]

To further complicate matters, analysis of tumors from people with schwannomatosis has revealed that multiple types of genetic alterations occur on chromosome 22, usually, but not always, in the same vicinity as the *NF2* gene.[7,8] This has led researchers to speculate that loss of some other tumor-suppressor gene, perhaps combined with loss of the *NF2* gene, may somehow cause schwannomatosis.[8] Another theory is that a structural element that makes the chromosome more susceptible to damage (or less easily repaired) may be at work. Normally chromosomes are separated and then recombined in an orderly fashion as cells divide to form new cells. A defect in this process can cause complete loss of genes or even part of a chromosome.[7,8]

In light of the conflicting data, some researchers theorize that any one of several different pathological mechanisms may result in schwannomatosis. Moreover, the mechanism responsible for the familial version of the disorder may be different from the defect involved in sporadic cases. This view is supported by the fact that several other neurological disorders are caused by one or more biological defects. One example is amyotrophic lateral sclerosis (ALS or "Lou Gehrig's" disease), which causes progressive motor deterioration. Although a gene responsible for the familial version of ALS was identified in 1993, subsequent research has shown that most sporadic cases develop because of some other biological insult, alone or in combination with others.

◆ Clinical Features

The defining clinical feature of schwannomatosis is the development of multiple schwannomas, and the dominant symptom is pain. Schwannomas are slow-growing benign tumors that do not turn malignant. Although solitary schwannomas may develop in the general population, whenever more than one such tumor develops, NF2 or schwannomatosis should be considered a possibility.

Along with other forms of neurofibromatosis, schwannomatosis is quite variable in its manifestation. There is no "typical" case. Some people develop many schwannomas; others develop only a few. Location and manifestations vary. Cranial schwannomas may be perceived as masses in the head or neck. Spinal schwannomas may cause severe pain before they are detected. Peripheral schwannomas may be clustered as masses and cause pain. Skin schwannomas may be mistaken for ordinary bumps or escape notice until diagnosis. In terms of appearance and cell type, the schwannomas associated with schwannomatosis are indistinguishable from those found in NF2 (see Chapter 10).

All people with schwannomatosis experience some degree of pain, but the intensity varies. Precise estimates of what proportion of patients experience what type of pain are hard to come by. In general, some people with schwannomatosis have such mild pain that they are never diagnosed with the disorder. Most people have significant pain, but it can be alleviated with medical or surgical treatment. In extreme but fortunately unusual cases, the pain is so severe and intractable that it is disabling. Those who endure this most severe manifestation of schwannomatosis cannot work or even function socially.

Pain can occur anywhere in the body and develops when a schwannoma enlarges, when it compresses nerve roots in the spine, or when it presses on adjacent tissue. Sometimes the pain is constant; at other times it is experienced whenever a sensitive area of the body is bumped or touched.

The pain associated with schwannomatosis is usually not accompanied by neurological deficit such as the hearing and balance losses seen in people with NF2. For this reason, the consulting physician may not immediately consider a tumor to be the cause of the pain, especially if no mass is evident upon physical examination. As a result, people with schwannomatosis typically experience pain for several years before receiving a proper diagnosis.

Neurological symptoms, however, do develop in some people with schwannomatosis. The first symptoms experienced are numbness, tingling, or weakness in the extremities. They are usually caused by a growing spinal tumor that compresses a portion of the spinal cord, but they may also be caused by a large peripheral schwannoma. Often the symptoms can be alleviated by removing the tumor surgically. Sometimes the tumor grows back or is inoperable, resulting in permanent loss of function.

One out of three people with schwannomatosis develops tumors in only one part of the body, for example, on one side of the body or in one limb.[5,9] It is not yet clear whether this is a subtype or a mosaic form of schwannomatosis. In the mosaic form the genetic defect occurs during prenatal development, and therefore it governs only part of the body (see Chapter 4).

◆ Guidelines for Diagnosis

Diagnostic criteria have been proposed for schwannomatosis and are provided in Table **12–1**. One challenge in diagnosis is to determine whether a person's pain is caused by schwannoma growth or has developed for some other reason. A second challenge is to rule out other forms of neurofibromatosis. It is usually easy to distinguish schwannomatosis from NF1; ruling out NF2 may take longer. To confirm a diagnosis, it may be

Table 12–1   Proposed Diagnostic Criteria for Schwannomatosis

Definite Schwannomatosis	Presumptive or Probable Schwannomatosis
Two or more pathologically proven schwannomas *plus*	Two or more pathologically proven schwannomas without symptoms of eighth nerve dysfunction when older than age 30 *or*
Lack of radiographic evidence of vestibular nerve tumor when older than age 18	Two or more pathologically proven schwannomas in an anatomically limited distribution (single limb or segment of spine) without symptoms of eighth nerve dysfunction, at any age

Adapted from Jacoby LB, Jones D, Davis K, et al. Molecular analysis of the *NF2* tumor-suppressor gene in schwannomatosis. Am J Hum Genet 1997;61:1301, with permission.

necessary to order a magnetic resonance imaging (MRI) scan of a suspected tumor and to analyze biopsied tissue.

Medical History

The medical history should include a review of the person's overall health with special attention given to symptoms that may indicate a diagnosis of schwannomatosis. Because the presenting symptom is usually pain, many of the questions asked to establish a medical history focus on when the pain first developed, whether it is episodic or chronic, and whether it may be caused by something other than a tumor. The patient should mention any injury, illness, or infection that occurred before the pain. It is important to describe as fully as possible the pain experienced, noting the precise location in the body where it occurs. Does the pain occur in only one part of the body or are there multiple locations? Is the pain more noticeable at one time of the day? Do external factors such as light or certain foods trigger the pain? All of these questions are necessary because pain is a poorly understood phenomenon, and there are many conditions that may cause pain (see Chapter 14).

If neurofibromatosis is suspected, additional questions may be posed to help the physician decide whether the patient has NF1, NF2, or schwannomatosis. The patient should be asked about café-au-lait spots, freckling, skin bumps and tender subcutaneous masses, when these features were first noticed, and whether and how they have changed over time. Any abnormalities in vision, hearing, balance, and learning should be discussed.

Family Medical History

Schwannomatosis is a genetic disorder, but it is not yet clear which gene causes it and how the disorder is inherited. Some researchers report that schwannomatosis sometimes skips generations (known medically as incomplete penetrance).[7] It is also not clear whether those people who inherit schwannomatosis experience the same manifestations as their relatives.

Given the uncertainties about the genetic transmission of schwanno-matosis, it is possible that a person with multiple schwannomas may have relatives with a mild and previously undiagnosed case of schwannomato-sis or even NF2. A person suspected of having schwannomatosis should be asked about the medical history of members of an extended family tree. This includes first-degree relatives (parents, siblings, children), second-degree relatives (grandparents, aunts, uncles, cousins), and more distant relations (great-grandparents, great-aunts and uncles, and descendants of second-degree relatives). If any relatives were diagnosed with NF1 or NF2, or experienced any unexplained pain or neurological symptoms, this should be noted and confirmed through medical records and direct physical examination whenever possible.

Physical Examination

The physical examination should include extra attention to the area of the body where the patient is experiencing pain. Schwannomas are encapsu-lated tumors, and sometimes are palpable, especially when located on peripheral nerves close to the surface of the skin. Spinal and cranial nerve schwannomas are not palpable, but may be suggested by a patient's de-scription of pain. Imaging studies of the related painful area may then be ordered to identify what may be causing the pain.

To rule out NF1 and NF2, the physical examination should include an assessment of features associated with both of these disorders. The skin should be examined for café-au-lait spots, freckling and neurofibromas (as-sociated with NF1; see Chapter 5), and schwannomas (suggestive of both NF2 and schwannomatosis; see Chapter 10). The physical examination may also include basic neurological, ophthalmologic, and auditory evaluations. This might entail an assessment of balance and coordination (Chapters 5 and 10), cataracts and retinal abnormalities (Chapter 10), hearing (Chapter 10), and an examination of the eyes for Lisch nodules (Chapter 5).

Medical Tests

Currently there are no blood or genetic tests to determine whether some-one has schwannomatosis. The diagnosis is confirmed with a combination of tissue analysis and imaging tests.

Pathological confirmation that a tumor is a schwannoma is estab-lished by a microscopic examination of excised tissue. Pathologically, schwannomas are homogeneous tumors because they consist predominantly of Schwann cells rather than the mix of cell types found in neurofibromas.

Cranial MRI of the eighth cranial nerve, described in Chapter 10, is a crucial step in determining correct diagnosis in someone with two or more pathologically confirmed schwannomas. If the cranial MRI reveals the presence of unilateral or bilateral vestibular schwannomas, the diagnosis is NF2. If no vestibular schwannomas are detected, follow-up screening depends on the patient's age and other symptoms. Although the proposed diagnostic criteria for schwannomatosis suggest that cranial MRI screening can be relaxed at age 18 years,[7] additional screening may be worthwhile inasmuch as some people develop vestibular schwannomas in their 20s and even later[4] (see differential diagnosis below).

Spinal MRI (Figs. **12–1** and **12–2**) is appropriate for anyone suspected of having schwannomatosis who is experiencing pain or numbness that might be explained by tumors pressing on nerve roots. Pain and other

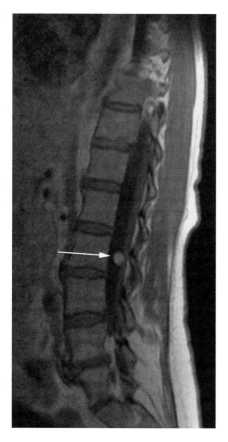

Figure 12–1 Magnetic resonance imaging (MRI) shows a schwannoma in the spinal column of a patient with schwannomatosis. (Courtesy of Carina Hirvela, M.D., and Ake Bodestedt, M.D., Uppsala University Hospital, Sweden, with permission.)

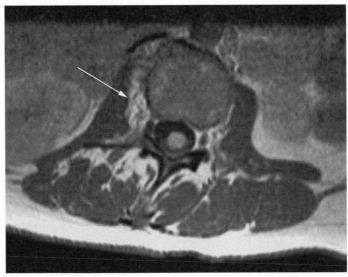

Figure 12–2   MRI taken from a different angle reveals the same schwannoma seen in Fig. 12–1. (Courtesy of Carina Hirvela, M.D., and Ake Bodestedt, M.D., Uppsala University Hospital, Sweden, with permission.)

symptoms may result in the back or the extremities, depending on the location of the tumor.

Additional imaging studies of other areas of the body (Figs. **12–3** and **12–4**) are appropriate when symptoms indicate a tumor may be located elsewhere in the body such as the chest, abdomen, or extremities.

◆ Differential Diagnosis

Schwannomatosis is most often confused with NF2. The easiest way to distinguish the two disorders is to determine whether or not the person has unilateral or bilateral vestibular schwannomas in addition to two or more pathologically confirmed schwannomas located elsewhere. This is most challenging during childhood and adolescence. Some manifestations of schwannomatosis, such as dermal and spinal schwannomas, are consistent with a diagnosis of NF2 and may precede the development of vestibular schwannomas. For that reason, people under age 30 suspected of having schwannomatosis should be monitored periodically for hearing loss and the development of vestibular schwannomas to rule out NF2.

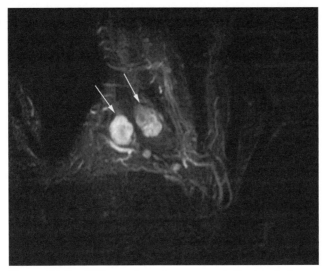

Figure 12–3 MRI reveals a schwannoma in the hand of a patient with schwannomatosis. (Courtesy of Carina Hirvela, M.D., and Ake Bodestedt, M.D., Uppsala University Hospital, Sweden, with permission.)

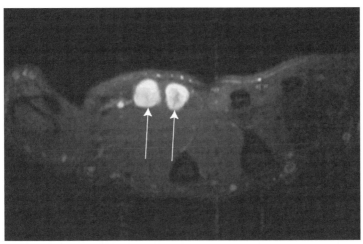

Figure 12–4 MRI taken from a different angle reveals the same schwannoma seen in Fig. 12–3. (Courtesy of Carina Hirvela, M.D., and Ake Bodestedt, M.D., Uppsala University Hospital, Sweden, with permission.)

Several clinical features help to distinguish schwannomatosis from NF1 and NF2, even before medical tests are ordered. The first feature is pain. People with NF1 and NF2 may experience episodic or chronic pain as a result of tumor growth, but it is not usually what prompts them to seek medical help and is not considered a defining manifestation for either disorder. People with schwannomatosis, on the other hand, often first seek medical help because of severe episodic and/or chronic pain, rather than a neurological deficit relating to vision or hearing loss, as is typical of NF1 and NF2. Second, though NF1 and NF2 usually present as generalized rather than mosaic disorders, that is not the case in schwannomatosis. A significant proportion of people with this disorder—about one in three—develop tumors only in one part of the body. Third, people with schwannomatosis do not develop other types of tumors associated with NF1 and NF2, including neurofibromas, meningiomas, ependymomas, and astrocytomas. Nor do they develop Lisch nodules and optic gliomas seen in NF1 or cataracts and other eye abnormalities seen in NF2. If any of these manifestations develop in a person found to have multiple skin tumors, a diagnosis of schwannomatosis should be ruled out.

◆ Management

Once a diagnosis of schwannomatosis is confirmed, management consists of surgery or medication to relieve pain, followed by ongoing monitoring and further intervention as needed.[4,5] Because schwannomatosis is rare and only recently has been recognized as a distinct disorder, there is no consensus about what screening tests should be ordered and how often. A complete MRI of the spine with contrast is usually performed as part of the initial evaluation. Periodic follow-up visits to a physician, preferably at a specialty clinic with expertise in neurofibromatosis, are recommended. Most clinicians agree that if schwannomas are detected during the initial examination and imaging tests, follow-up screening is necessary only if pain or other symptoms develop or change in intensity.

There is no established treatment protocol for schwannomatosis. In general, surgery is the mainstay of treatment to relieve pain because it removes the causative tumor. Many people experience considerable pain relief following surgery. Although the exact surgical technique depends on the location of the schwannoma, the goal is to completely remove the tumor while preserving the nerve if possible so that function is not imperiled. Complete resection of the tumor is not always possible, however, and if any fragments of a schwannoma remain the tumor may grow back, although the rate of growth is usually slow.

Prophylactic surgery to prevent pain is not recommended. A schwannoma may never cause pain and should not be removed simply because it is detected on an imaging scan. Any surgical procedure involves risks and should be considered only when these are outweighed by the potential benefits of intervention.

If surgery fails to provide relief or carries too many risks, an overall pain management strategy should be developed. The elements of a pain management plan are described in Chapter 14. In general, people with schwannomatosis experience such severe pain that a multiprong, whole-body approach is the only one that will work. The goal is to identify triggers that can worsen and amplify pain. Stress and lack of adequate sleep, for instance, are two common factors that significantly worsen pain. Individual patients may have specific pain triggers. Patients should think about, and doctors should ask about, what circumstances seem to make pain subside and what circumstances make it worse. This helps identify pain triggers for that individual person. A consultation with a physical or occupational therapist may further help to identify what activities or body postures aggravate pain. An individualized strategy to counter pain triggers can then be developed. A person whose pain worsens with stress, for instance, may benefit from techniques such as relaxation exercises, deep breathing, and practices such as Tai Chi that involve gentle movements.

In most cases, people with schwannomatosis also require treatment with medications to control pain. People whose pain is mild may require only the occasional over-the-counter pain reliever, such as aspirin or acetaminophen. If a person with schwannomatosis is taking an over-the-counter pain reliever every day, however, a more aggressive approach is probably necessary. To develop an individual strategy, the patient should work with a specialist at an NF clinic or seek a consultation at a pain management clinic (Chapter 14 discusses how to find a specialist). Medications that calm nerves or subdue the signaling between nerves are often effective because they prevent pain from occurring in the first place. Many of these medications also aid sleep, thereby preventing inadequate sleep as a pain trigger. Sometimes medications are prescribed in combination to make them more effective (see Chapter 14).

◆ Genetic Counseling

People with schwannomatosis who want to have children, or who became parents before being diagnosed, often wonder about the genetic risk to offspring. Unfortunately, genetic counseling is difficult to provide for anyone diagnosed with schwannomatosis because not enough is yet known about the mechanism responsible for this disorder. There are clearly defined instances where schwannomatosis is transmitted from one generation to another in an apparently dominant genetic manner, with offspring facing a 50/50 chance of inheriting the disorder. The far more common situation, however, involves sporadic occurrence. Until the causative mechanism is identified, physicians can provide little guidance to patients about risk of passing schwannomatosis on to offspring.

In general, in people with schwannomatosis who have no family history of the disorder, confirmed by examining an extended family tree, the risk of passing the disorder on to offspring is apparently low, but not zero. The risk of passing the disorder on to grandchildren under these circumstances is also low but not zero. Those patients who do have a family history face a higher, but as yet unquantified, chance of passing the disorder on. More will be learned when the gene or mechanism causing schwannomatosis is identified.

◆ The Personal Perspective

Marcy H.: "For many years before I was diagnosed, I had horrible pain. I went to doctors, and they diagnosed me with sacroiliitis [severe pain in the lower back area] and spondylitis [an inflammation of the vertebrae]. The pain first started when I was pregnant with my daughter, who was my first child. I developed a horrible pain down my sciatic nerve. I think that the doctors would have ordered an MRI for a man with the same symptoms, but they dismissed my concerns as 'hormonal' because I was pregnant.

"About five years later, I went to a doctor who thought I had a swollen lymph node. First he put me on antibiotics, but the problem didn't go away. And I knew something was weird about it. Because I said, 'When you press on it, there's pain,' he sent me to a surgeon who performed a needle biopsy. The surgeon called my internist; they thought I had cancer. When they operated, they found a tumor in my brachial plexus.

"I finally diagnosed myself. After I had surgery, I saw an article about neurofibromatosis on a bulletin board while I was walking down the hallway of a neurosurgical ward. I read the article, and I said to my husband, 'This is what I have.' My doctors finally diagnosed me, first as having neurofibromatosis. This was before schwannomatosis even had a name.

"Once I had a semi-diagnosis, the doctor advised having an MRI twice a year, then yearly, and now it's once every three years. I usually feel pain before anything shows up on an MRI. I've had at least 38 tumors removed in five years.

"The pain is excruciating. Any pain I've had postsurgery is a '1,' but the daily pain of living with schwannomatosis is a '10.' I can't sleep much at night because of the pain, and I have very little appetite. I'm an 89-pound, 4-foot-11-inch weakling. The pain is so severe that I feel nauseous and don't want to eat.

"There's no family history of this disorder. I've had a genetic analysis of my blood, and the doctors found an abnormality on two different genes. They also analyzed my parents' blood. The doctors think my case is spontaneous. After I found out that this could be genetic, I had my kids checked by a neurologist. I felt so guilty; I wanted to put my mind at rest. I don't want to scare them or make them think they have it. So far they're fine."

References

1. Shishiba T, Niimura M, Ohtsuka F, Tsuru N. Multiple cutaneous neurilemomas as a skin manifestation of neurilemomatosis. J Am Acad Dermatol 1984;10:744–754
2. Seppala MT, Sainio MA, Haltia MJ, Kinnunen JJ, Setala KH, Jaaskelainen JE. Multiple schwannomas: schwannomatosis or neurofibromatosis type 2? J Neurosurg 1998;89:36–41
3. Antinheimo J, Sankila R, Carpen O, Pukkala E, Sainio M, Jaaskelainen J. Population-based analysis of sporadic and type 2 neurofibromatosis-associated meningiomas and schwannomas. Neurology 2000;54:71–76
4. Evans DG, Mason S, Huson SM, Ponder M, Harding AE, Strachan T. Spinal and cutaneous schwannomatosis is a variant form of type 2 neurofibromatosis: a clinical and molecular study. J Neurol Neurosurg Psychiatry 1997;62:361–366
5. MacCollin M, Woodfin W, Kronn D, Short MP. Schwannomatosis: a clinical and pathologic study. Neurology 1996;46:1072–1079
6. Ruggieri M, Huson SM. The neurofibromatoses: an overview. Ital J Neurol Sci 1999;20:89–108
7. Jacoby LB, Jones D, Davis K, et al. Molecular analysis of the NF2 tumor-suppressor gene in schwannomatosis. Am J Hum Genet 1997;61:1293–1302
8. MacCollin M, Willett C, Heinrich B, et al. Familial schwannomatosis: exclusion of the NF2 locus as the germline event. Neurology 2003;60:1968–1974
9. Verma RR, Khan MT, Davies AM, Mangham DC, Grimer RJ. Subperiosteal schwannomas of the femur. Skeletal Radiol 2002;31:422–425

13

Psychosocial Impact of Neurofibromatosis

Neurofibromatosis (NF) has a psychosocial impact that consists of psychological, social, economic, and quality-of-life issues. Psychosocial issues pervade the life of not only the individual with neurofibromatosis, but also the spouse, family members, and other loved ones. This chapter explores the psychosocial impact of neurofibromatosis and suggests coping strategies and resources.

Although the psychosocial aspects of neurofibromatosis have not been studied as extensively as the disorder's physical manifestations, research and personal accounts of people who have NF have helped to identify common areas of concern and typical coping mechanisms.[1-5] Psychosocial impact of neurofibromatosis is lifelong and may change over time. An adolescent may be most concerned with physical appearance; an adult may be more concerned about marriage, childbearing, and career choices. Parents of a child with neurofibromatosis may struggle with feelings of guilt, grief, and worry; unaffected siblings may resent the attention given to the child with the disorder.

Although many of the psychosocial issues discussed are painful and challenging, most people with neurofibromatosis are happy and well adjusted. In interviews, many say that dealing with the disorder has helped them to become resourceful, resilient, better communicators, and more appreciative of the good things in life. They have dealt with negative emotions and experiences, but they have learned how to acknowledge the pain and move beyond it. They cherish the many positive aspects of their lives, focus on the important things, live and enjoy life fully.

◆ The Impact of Diagnosis

People react to a diagnosis of neurofibromatosis in different ways, but it almost always provokes strong emotions and presents significant psychological challenges. There are many reasons for this, chief among them fear of the unknown. In neurofibromatosis, this fear has two dimensions: fear of what manifestations will eventually develop, and fear of how severe those manifestations will be. Most people with neurofibromatosis face the prospect of living their lives with uncertainty about what the future holds in terms of their health and ability to function. Other emotional triggers include changes in physical appearance, feelings of isolation, and experiencing stigma. Certain emotions may subside and then resurge as new features of neurofibromatosis 1 (NF1) develop, or as neurofibromatosis complicates significant life choices such as the decision whether to have children. Given all these factors, neurofibromatosis imposes an enormous emotional burden on individuals and families.

Emotions

When people receive a diagnosis of a chronic disorder such as neurofibromatosis, they are likely to experience intense emotions. Some psychologists believe the emotional reactions to diagnosis of a serious illness are similar to those experienced at the end of life, which were first described by the Swiss psychiatrist Elisabeth Kübler-Ross in her book, *On Death and Dying*. Kübler-Ross identified five stages of grief: denial, anger, bargaining, depression, and acceptance.[6] These emotions may or may not occur in the order Kübler-Ross proposed; people may also cycle back and forth between emotions before finally accepting the reality of neurofibromatosis. At the same time, friends and loved ones may go through a similar process. All of this can make for an emotional maelstrom, to say the least, especially because people go through various stages of the process at different times, and the process itself is not always linear.

When first diagnosed, a person (or the parents, in the case of a child) may feel only shock and numbing disbelief. This "transient denial" is a form of emotional self-protection, to enable the person to cope in stages. Usually the denial stage passes, but it can become dangerous if it persists and prevents someone from seeking medical attention when appropriate.

As time passes, denial may take the form of being optimistic, not thinking about the diagnosis much, and dealing with problems as they arise.

Anger may be next. It is common for people to demand: Why me? How could this happen? People going through this stage may become angry over small things, lash out at a spouse or significant other, or find fault with doctors and medical staff. Anger is a difficult emotion to experience, not only for the person who has NF, but for those with whom he or she interacts, yet it may be necessary as part of the healing process. Anger becomes destructive, however, if it becomes chronic and ingrained.

Bargaining may take the form of trying to find strategies that will preclude new health concerns. A person going through this stage may adopt a new diet in an effort to remain healthy or take pains to avoid exposure to environmental toxins. Such strategies often provide a sense of control, whereas the diagnosis has made the person feel completely out of control.

Depression may occur when the person with NF acknowledges the reality of diagnosis but is profoundly sad about it. Typically during this stage, he or she will feel tired, irritable, and even victimized. Once again, the issue to be concerned about is duration; if symptoms persist continuously for 2 weeks or more, the individual may need medical help from a clinical psychologist or psychiatrist.[7]

Interpersonal Stress

Given the difficult emotions that may be engendered by a diagnosis of NF1 or NF2, it's not surprising that the person may also experience difficulties dealing with other people. Family members and spouses or partners may or may not react in a supportive way, as they struggle with their own emotions. At the same time, the person who receives a diagnosis may have to start meeting with several new people, including physicians and other medical staff, insurance representatives, and, in the case of a child, with school officials and administrators. If multiple medical appointments are required, transportation and child care may also pose challenges.

Intellectual Stress

Most people who receive a diagnosis do not have medical training, and even those who do may not be familiar with NF1 or NF2. The person who receives the diagnosis is trying to grasp a lot of new information and to make informed medical decisions, while simultaneously dealing with the emotions described above. Intellectual stress can be especially burdensome in the first days, weeks, and even months following a diagnosis. This type of stress tends to abate with time, as people find information they trust, absorb the details, and grow more familiar with the condition.

Additional Stresses

Diagnosis never happens in a vacuum. The people it touches may be simultaneously trying to cope with financial difficulties, job pressures, marital strain or divorce, or have preexisting emotional difficulties such as depression. All of these factors may exacerbate the reactions mentioned earlier.

◆ Coping with a Diagnosis

The first step in accepting a diagnosis is to appreciate how difficult this may be, for all the reasons just described. Many of the early emotional reactions subside with time. In general, seek help for yourself or a loved one, or make a referral for a patient, when emotional states start to interfere with sleep, work, family life, and important daily routines.

Genetic counseling may also help to better clarify both the disorder and its implications for childbearing decisions. The amount and type of information provided depend on the age of the patient (see Chapter 4).

Whenever possible, physicians should offer patients written information about neurofibromatosis at the time of diagnosis. This should include information about the genetics of neurofibromatosis and the risk of passing the disorder on to children. If additional medical visits are necessary, or expert consultations required, names and contact information for the appropriate physicians should be provided at the time of diagnosis. It is a rare person who will remember every medical detail explained at the time of diagnosis, and patient information sheets or brochures help answer questions that occur once the person has gone home. [The National Neurofibromatosis Foundation (NNFF) has available several excellent brochures, books, and other materials. For more information, visit the NF Foundation Web site: www.nf.org.]

Patients can help themselves by obtaining as much information as they personally feel necessary. Some people prefer to rely on physicians, who can interpret the information for them. In some areas of the country, chapters of the NNFF provide regular meetings with programs presented by medical professionals. The person with NF has the opportunity not only to learn more about the disorder but also to meet other people who have it. In many cases this has provided the first occasion for a person to meet someone else who has NF. Chapters offer a way for individuals to take active part in the programs of the NNFF and thus contribute to its educational and research goals.

Support groups are sometimes available, which may be useful in providing emotional support and practical information about personal experience of others and local resources. Parents of newly diagnosed children who are interested in support groups should be aware of the substantial variability of severity of NF1. In a support group, they may meet parents or individuals who are dealing with severe complications of the disorder.

Finally, patients can help themselves by becoming active participants in their own care. Ask questions, seek second opinions as necessary, and keep track of medical visits and clinical findings. Sample forms for use in compiling information and keeping track of medical visits are included in Chapter 14.

◆ Talking About Neurofibromatosis

Talking with Children

Parents of children with neurofibromatosis are often concerned about when and how to explain the disorder to a child. Some general principles are helpful for parents in talking about neurofibromatosis with an affected child, unaffected siblings, or other children:

- Deal with your own emotions first.
- Don't explain everything at once. Answer questions as the child asks them and provide only information a child is ready to comprehend. Many parents find it helpful to handle the issue as they would questions about sex. Listen to the child and try to understand what he or she wants to know, answering one question at a time.
- Be honest, even if the vocabulary used is simple. Evasive answers will erode trust.
- Use the accurate words rather than euphemisms. Talk about neurofibromas or schwannomas, not just "bumps" and "boo-boos." (Otherwise the child may grow anxious whenever a normal bump or cut develops.)
- It's all right not to know all the answers. If uncertain about how to answer a question, tell the child you will check with a physician or other source to find the answer.

Telling Others

Adults with neurofibromatosis may struggle with when and how to tell others about the diagnosis. The decision may depend on how obvious the disorder is, whether disclosure is to friends, neighbors, work colleagues, or relatives, and on an individual's own sense of privacy.

- Divulge only what you feel comfortable sharing.
- Rehearse responses to difficult questions ahead of time. For example,

the word *tumor* is often interpreted as "cancer." *Benign growth* or *lesion* may be a better term.
- Be prepared to answer absurd, impolite, or personal questions. A common concern people have is whether neurofibromatosis is an infectious condition. Not many people understand the way genetic disorders are transmitted.

◆ Dealing with Ongoing Concerns

Challenges remain even after people come to accept a diagnosis of neurofibromatosis. Individuals and families may find themselves occasionally cycling back through a process of grief and acceptance as they confront the ongoing challenges of neurofibromatosis. Although individual experience varies, such challenges usually include some mix of issues described below.

Living with Uncertainty

Anyone who has had to wait to hear the results of a medical test knows how difficult it can be to deal with uncertainty about what the future holds. Most people with neurofibromatosis face this type of uncertainty every day of their lives. In all cases of NF1 and schwannomatosis, and in spontaneous cases of NF2, it is impossible to predict exactly what mix of symptoms will develop and how severe they will become. It is normal, in the face of such uncertainty, to feel anxious, worried, stressed, angry, and depressed. People with neurofibromatosis often say that having to cope with uncertainty is the most challenging aspect of their disorder.

Feelings of Isolation

It is common for people with any disorder to ask, "Why me?" This may occur not only at the time of diagnosis but also throughout life as different challenges arise. One can feel lonely and isolated in having a disorder like neurofibromatosis that people may be unfamiliar with, fear, or have misconceptions about. People may mistakenly believe they can "catch" neurofibromatosis and thus avoid someone with the disorder. Someone with neurofibromatosis may resent the fact that other people, even other family members, do not face similar challenges.

Changes in Physical Appearance

Neurofibromatosis has physical manifestations that may make the person with NF look "different" from other people. Such differences can pose enormous difficulty, especially in societies like the United States in which unrealistic norms for beauty are continually reinforced in the media. People with NF1 may worry about visible café-au-lait spots and dermal neurofibromas. They may be afraid that they will become disfigured, although most people with NF1 do not. People with all types of neurofibromatosis who develop visible tumors in the face, neck, arms, and trunk are especially vulnerable to feeling self-conscious about physical appearance. They feel it is necessary to wear clothing that covers the arms and trunk even though that might not be their style preference. The physical changes associated with neurofibromatosis pose more than just cosmetic challenges in that they can threaten a person's sense of self-esteem and security.

Stigma

The word *stigma* derives from the Greek word for a mark made with a sharp instrument. People with neurofibromatosis may indeed feel "marked," either physically or emotionally, by the disorder. Having to confront stigma is a fact of life for most people with neurofibromatosis. Such stigma may be as blatant as the taunts of schoolchildren or as subtle as someone in a shopping mall staring too long. It can include avoidance, ostracism, revulsion, rejection, fear of contagion, and lowered expectations. Stigma may also manifest as discrimination in the workplace and by insurance companies.

Problems Making Friends

In childhood and adolescence, people with neurofibromatosis may have trouble making and keeping friends. Sometimes other children make fun of a child with neurofibromatosis because of visible tumors or other physical differences. Repeated school absences to deal with doctor visits and medical treatments may prevent a child from keeping up with peers. The child may feel self-conscious about changing clothes for gym class or attending sleep-overs and pool parties. In NF1, learning disabilities and coexisting disorders like attention deficit hyperactivity disorder (ADHD) may require the child to attend special classes or take medication. The onset of early or late puberty may further distance the child from peers.

Concern About Intimate Relationships

As a person with neurofibromatosis matures, dating and marriage may become a concern. It is natural for any adolescent to be shy and awkward around the opposite sex, but this may be especially true of someone concerned about physical appearance or having to explain what a genetic disorder is. Adults with neurofibromatosis may struggle with when and how to tell people they're dating about the disorder because it will influence long-term decisions about marriage and childbearing.

Coping with a Lifelong Disorder

The neurofibromatoses are chronic disorders that pose different challenges at different stages of life. Coping with a lifelong disorder requires that a person find ways to continually adjust to and cope with new circumstances.

Challenges of a Genetic Disorder

A disorder that involves genetic transmission poses unique challenges to individuals and families. Parents of someone with neurofibromatosis may struggle with feelings of guilt and personal responsibility about "giving this" to a child, even if there is no family history of the disorder. Individuals with neurofibromatosis may struggle with the decision to marry and have biological children.

◆ Issues Affecting Families and Loved Ones

Neurofibromatosis is a disorder that engulfs the entire family. It can place strains on a marriage, as parents struggle to cope with multiple difficult and unexpected challenges: accepting the diagnosis, finding accurate information about neurofibromatosis, seeking knowledgeable health care providers, accommodating numerous doctor visits, dealing with learning disability and poor school performance, aiding the child's social development, and providing a supportive home for the child. Each partner in a marriage may have different coping methods: one may want to talk to "let off steam," while the other prefers to avoid the topic. Financial worries and concerns about the future of a child who has NF only further complicate matters. Guilt, however irrational from a scientific viewpoint, often plagues parents.

Unaffected siblings may resent the attention given to the child with neurofibromatosis or may feel "survivor's guilt" at having been spared. The child with NF may grow frustrated at having to face challenges others in the family do not face. If burdened with learning or physical disabilities, he or she may become discouraged at not being able to keep up with schoolmates, siblings, and other family members.

In spite of these challenges, parents and siblings can provide enormous support to a child who has NF by creating a family atmosphere of respect and acceptance. Most experts agree that it is best to treat a child with neurofibromatosis the same as any other child. Acknowledge that the child is facing unique challenges and emotions, but maintain the expectation that the child will achieve his or her full potential. As the child becomes an adult, encourage as much independence as possible.

It also helps to remember that all families experience good and bad times, but that the main point is to keep communicating. Families absorbed with neurofibromatosis may have to make a special effort to schedule family time and activities so that home life does not revolve around medical visits or other aspects of living with the disorder.

◆ Coping with Ongoing Concerns

Find Support

Some of the best advice about how to deal with the psychosocial aspects of neurofibromatosis has come from those who have it. The National Neurofibromatosis Foundation shares such information and provides support to people with neurofibromatosis and their families in a variety of ways. NF Foundation chapters are located across the country and may be able to provide a referral to a local support group. A newsletter, an online bulletin board, and a community chat room are available at the NF Foundation Web site: www.nf.org.

Take It a Day at a Time

People usually feel overwhelmed when they are trying to process too much information or make too many decisions at once. In neurofibromatosis, it is important to take the disorder one day at a time, and even one task or one decision at a time. If a doctor is concerned about a new symptom and orders a medical test, for instance, it may be more helpful to focus on the factors you can control than worry about an outcome you can't predict. Ask whether you will have to fast or do anything else in preparation for the test. Ask how long it will take and whether someone should accompany you. When will the results be known and, if necessary, when will treatment options be discussed? Whatever the issue, try to deal with the challenges that exist and try not to think of others that may develop at some point in the future.

Explore Creative Coping Methods

Everyone has a personal way of dealing with adversity. Some people like to gather as much information as possible; others avoid reading anything for fear of increasing their anxiety. Sometimes it helps to broaden your skills in this area by experimenting with other ways of coping, even if the methods don't appeal at first. You never known until you try. Options for coping include physical activity to work off emotional "steam," relaxation techniques such as meditation and deep breathing, and distractions such as meeting with friends or going to a movie.

Tell People What You Need from Them

Don't be afraid to ask for help and support when you need it. Be specific. Even loved ones and the best of friends may not understand what you need and may end up doing exactly what you wish they wouldn't do. Different people offer different strengths. Learn which people you can turn to for emotional support, practical advice, and financial help. It is rare to find one person who can provide all of this.

Become an Active Participant in Your Health Care

You know your own body, or your child, better than anyone. Become familiar with your overall health profile so that you can articulate changes to your health care provider. Ask questions if you don't understand, request supplementary educational material, and seek out your own sources of information on the Internet or in the library. Don't be afraid to question treatment recommendations or ask for a second opinion if you have concerns. Remember that medicine is always evolving. Ask about new treatment options or research studies that may be appropriate (see Chapter 15). For news about research findings, clinical trials, and new treatments, visit the NF Foundation Web site: www.nf.org.

Explore Alternative Therapies

Mention alternative medicine and most people think of herbs sold in a health food store. Yet alternative therapies include a wide variety of non-medical approaches to fostering emotional and physical health. Relaxation techniques such as deep breathing and meditation help some people with neurofibromatosis to ease anxiety. Others benefit from yoga (a series of gentle stretches combined with meditation), tai chi (slow dance-like movements to stimulate the flow of life energy), and reiki (in which a practitioner channels spiritual energy to promote healing).

Cultivate Faith and Spirituality

Some people with neurofibromatosis find that participating in religious services or some other type of spiritual observation helps to promote overall health and well-being. Prayer, faith, and spirituality can be sources of enormous strength.

Get Professional Help When Appropriate

Although everyone occasionally feels down or gets the blues, it is important to seek professional help if these feelings become pronounced or persist for too long. If someone with neurofibromatosis is depressed, fatigued, has trouble sleeping, or unable to concentrate almost every day for a 2-week period, the cause could be major depression.[7] If these symptoms, or any significant change in mood and/or energy level occur, it is best to seek medical attention from a clinical psychologist or psychiatrist.

◆ The Personal Perspective

Nancy B: "I have concerns about the future. NF1 is unpredictable in the course it can take. It probably won't get bad, but it's always in the back of my mind that it could get worse. Watching my twin sister, who also has NF1, go through her recent operation to remove a plexiform neurofibroma churned up lots of emotions."

Porter C.: "Sometimes people point, laugh, and stare and call me names. I wish that they would ask questions. When children ask, some parents try to stop them and I say, 'No, let him ask.'

"I now have reiki treatments once a week. It's an ancient Japanese healing technique that involves hands-on healing. My cat is interested in it and recently jumped up on the table and stretched out on my back. He wanted a treatment too.

"I don't feel sorry for myself. Positive thinking helps. I was blessed with parents who had a lot to do with my attitude. A good sense of humor helps. Life was meant to be lived, and I'm not going to live in a closet because someone doesn't like my looks."

Diane D.: "The emotional impact of NF1 is proving to be more challenging than the medical aspect. Knowing that most of the medical symptoms of NF1 can be managed, I think we can handle anything that comes medically. If tumors develop, they are usually benign. It's the emotional part of the day-to-day challenges for Julie that is so difficult. The problems making friends, the struggling in school, problems learning—that's what is so hard."

Dolores G.: "You know, there's always such a concern about 'whose fault is it.' My parents blamed my husband, and my husband's family blamed me. When I was diagnosed it took the heat off my mother-in-law and put a terrible load of guilt on my parents, especially my mother. I remember exactly where we were when I told my parents I did not have NF. We were in the hospital, in the cafeteria, and it was Susan and her dad and me, and my mom and dad. We were sitting there, eating with Susan. And I told my mother that I was 'de-diagnosed,' to use my terminology. As I told my mother about this, you could see this burden being physically lifted from her. It was amazing. My parents adored Susan and would have done anything for her. But just knowing that it wasn't her fault, that she didn't have it, made such a difference in my mother.

"My husband and I did have pressure, yet we could work it out on our own. But it was tough on our other kids. I don't think we neglected the other kids, and they tell me now that we didn't, but there was always this illness that was like a cloud over our heads. It's not that one person in the family has NF; it's that the whole family has NF."

Adam G.: "I never let NF2 affect me. I never saw NF2 as an excuse and I never saw it as a reason that I should not be able to achieve as much, so I think my attitude has helped. When I was younger, in elementary school, there were kids who made fun of me. But even at that age, I realized these kids didn't know what they were talking about. I've done a lot of speaking at school assemblies. My class knows me well. I'm secretary of my class. So they know there's a lot more to me than that I'm blind in one eye and deaf in one ear."

Marcy H.: "Before I received a diagnosis, it was very difficult. I was in so much pain. And when you're in pain, you become hard to live with. It can be very hard for a couple, and a family, before there is a diagnosis.

"Today my husband is incredibly supportive, although he had a hard time adjusting to this. Men like to fix things, and he can't fix this. It's probably as difficult for the family as it is for the patient. The spouse is dealing with something that he has no clue about. You look fine and you're supposed to act fine. The family can become exhausted from it. They get sick of hearing about it.

"My husband and I both see a psychologist. My psychologist works with people who have pain disorders. I'd advise others to seek out psychological help with a therapist who is willing to talk with both the individual and the family. You want to work with someone who tries to keep the couple together."

Martha L.: "When I was diagnosed, no one really knew then, or even now, how NF2 will affect each individual. I was scared, angry, and devastated, not knowing what the future would hold, and knowing that I would lose my hearing. The biggest challenge I have faced is accepting what is wrong with me and trying to explain to people what NF2 is and why this happened. People are afraid of the unknown, and NF is just that. One of my biggest concerns now is that a tumor will take away my ability to be independent.

"Having NF has taught me a lot about life, and to be grateful for it. I've always loved my family and friends, but having a disease makes you appreciate the things closest to you even more. I know when this all started, and sometimes even now, I would get depressed or sad and think, Why me? My parents and my sisters have been there for me since this all started. I was lucky enough to meet my husband, to whom I've been married for 10 years. It's been my husband who has had to see me at my saddest and most depressed times, but he's been right there holding my hand every step of the way. I truly believe without these wonderful people in my life, I don't think I could be the way I am today. NF has made my body weaker in some ways, but it has made my heart and my love of life much stronger."

Tamra M.: "My friends in school have a good idea about what NF is. I've done a few presentations on it in science and health. People have been very supportive. My high school has been really great compared to other schools my friends with NF have told me about. There's compassion. When I was in the hospital, everyone signed a card, even people I didn't know."

References

1. Psychosocial Aspects of the Neurofibromatoses: Impact on the Individual, Impact on the Family. Jane Novak Pugh Conference Series, vol. 3. New York: National Neurofibromatosis Foundation; 1992
2. Ablon J. Living with Genetic Disorder: The Impact of Neurofibromatosis 1. Westport, CT: Auburn House; 1999
3. Messner RL, Gardner S, Messner MR. Neurofibromatosis—an international enigma: a framework for nursing. Cancer Nurs 1985;8:314–322
4. Messner RL, Messner MR, Lewis SJ. Neurofibromatosis: a familial and family disorder. J Neurosurg Nurs 1985;17:221–228
5. Messner RL, Smith MN. Neurofibromatosis: relinquishing the masks; a quest for quality of life. J Adv Nurs 1986;11:459–464
6. Kübler-Ross E. On Death and Dying. New York: Scribner; 1997
7. American Psychiatric Association. Diagnostic and Statistical Manual of Mental Disorders. 4th ed. Washington, DC: American Psychiatric Association; 1994:320–327

14

Practical and Quality-of-Life Issues

This chapter focuses on the major practical and quality-of-life aspects of living with neurofibromatosis (NF). Logistical challenges include coordinating multiple medical visits, navigating the insurance system, and identifying resources to fill gaps in care. Economic challenges include out-of-pocket expenses on health care, lost wages and earnings due to medical absences, and job discrimination. Some people with neurofibromatosis must also contend with pain, a significant medical challenge that may require a combination of management strategies.

◆ Finding Knowledgeable Doctors

Finding a physician who is knowledgeable about neurofibromatosis can present a major challenge. Many people with neurofibromatosis have encountered at least one health care professional who provided outdated or erroneous information and advice.

The easiest way to identify a doctor familiar with neurofibromatosis is through referral. Although finding a specialist in neurofibromatosis is usually the best choice, it is also possible to receive excellent care from a general practice physician or a specialist in genetic disorders. Begin by asking your own pediatrician or primary care physician for a recommendation in your area. Even if your own doctor is not able to identify a specialist, he or she may be able to connect you with someone who can. The NF Foundation is another excellent source of information and referrals. The NF Foundation's Clinical Care Advisory Board establishes standards for diagnosis and treatment and maintains a list of specialized clinical care centers in the U.S. (This list is available at the NF Foundation Web site: www.nf.org.) Local NF Foundation chapters or affiliates represent yet another source of valuable information. Participants can share advice about doctors who have experience with NF in their city or state.

◆ Coordinating Care

It can be overwhelming to deal with the physical and psychosocial aspects of neurofibromatosis while simultaneously trying to navigate the medical system. Typically people with neurofibromatosis must schedule multiple medical visits and surgical consults—often at different institutions and perhaps even in different parts of the country—and then keep track of results and follow-up appointments. For parents of children with the disorder, an added challenge is dealing with the school system, especially if the child has one or more learning disabilities and a behavioral disorder such as attention deficit disorder (ADD) or attention deficit hyperactivity disorder (ADHD).

Some people seem to juggle all this effortlessly. For those who don't, the following strategies may help to better coordinate care.

Identify a Case Manager

When multiple health care providers are involved, it may help to identify one as the "case manager" or "quarterback" who will coordinate paperwork and communication between providers. Often the case manager is a physician. At other times, a nurse, social worker, or genetic counselor may play this role. The choice of case manager depends in part on the hospital or medical office that provides care, for different providers have different ways of organizing their practices. It may also depend on whom the individual with neurofibromatosis feels most comfortable with. Be aware that health insurers do not usually cover case management, so that the medical professional assuming this role will have to make time for it on top of other duties.

Assign a Family Point Person

Another way to eliminate confusion is to assign one person in the family as point person for communicating with medical professionals and keeping track of health care visits and other medical details. The individual may be the person who has neurofibromatosis, a spouse, parents, or even siblings and other relatives. Whoever is chosen should be organized, good at communicating, and comfortable with the medical system. It is less confusing all around if one person handles medical communications and logistics. This cuts down on the amount of information repeated or lost and helps to ensure follow-up.

Get Organized

Keep a record of medical visits, tests performed, the results, and recommended follow-up. Although any medical office keeps records of patient visits, people with neurofibromatosis generally have multiple medical records located at different institutions. The best way to ensure that all the information is located in one place is to keep personal files. Patients can ask for copies of reports and test results to supplement their own notes. Sample forms to keep track of medical information are shown in Tables **14–1**, **14–2**, and **14–3** (see end of chapter). Some people prefer to organize the various data by file; others put them in three-ring binders. There is no one-size-fits-all approach to getting organized, but it is important to find a method that works for you.

◆ Medical Privacy Protections

Every patient has a right to confidentiality concerning medical information. The federal Health Insurance Portability and Accountability Act of 1996 (HIPAA) requires that the federal government set uniform standards for patient confidentiality. The Department of Health and Human Services issued a HIPAA Privacy Rule that went into effect in April 2003 and significantly widened privacy protections, applying them to medical offices, hospitals, and insurance companies. Under the HIPAA Privacy Rule, health care providers may release medical information about a patient only when that patient provides written permission to do so, except when related to providing treatment, obtaining payment from an insurer, or contacting the patient about appointments or providing the patient with medical information. Certain other exceptions are also allowed. For instance, medical providers may share the information with medical colleagues involved in a patient's care and with designated family members. The Privacy Rule authorizes patients to view their medical records at any time and request limits on how that information may be shared with others.

The laws regarding medical privacy are complicated and each health care provider or institution may have its own policies regarding confidentiality. If medical privacy is a concern, ask the institution for a copy of its confidentiality policy. To learn more about the HIPAA Privacy Rule, contact the Office for Civil Rights in the U.S. Department of Health and Human Services.

◆ Health Insurance

Health insurance is often a big concern for people with neurofibromatosis and their loved ones. The patchwork nature of the health insurance industry, with a variety of plans and insurers available, only adds to the anxiety. To make the process of finding health insurance easier, people with neurofibromatosis should familiarize themselves with several issues.

Types of Plans Available

Most people in the United States obtain health insurance through their employers. People with neurofibromatosis cannot legally be excluded from such employer-sponsored group plans, but may have to wait for a specified period before having access to certain benefits if the policy has a preexisting condition clause (discussed below). Assuming the company offers family as well as individual coverage, an employee's dependent child with neurofibromatosis is covered until early adulthood (age varies depending on the plan).

Self-employed people, and those whose employers do not offer health insurance, may obtain individual coverage through a local Chamber of Commerce, insurance broker, or membership in a professional association. People living on limited incomes and those who are disabled may be eligible for a government program such as Medicare or Medicaid. Many hospitals also provide financial assistance to patients and families unable to meet all or part of their bills, although eligibility criteria and application procedures vary. Ask your health care provider about this resource or contact the institution's patient relations office.

Indemnity plans pay for care on a fee-for-service basis and allow a patient the most freedom in choosing health care providers and services. Premiums for such plans tend to be high and few employers today offer them.

Self-insured plans are funded and administered by the employer. Large companies with thousands of employees tend to offer such plans, which are not always subject to state regulation and therefore may not provide all of the benefits available through indemnity and managed-care plans.

Managed care plans encompass a variety of options offering some mix of choice and cost control. Managed care plans are the most common type of health insurance coverage available today.

- *Health maintenance organizations (HMOs)* require patients to choose a primary care physician who acts as a "gatekeeper" for referral to specialists.
- *Preferred provider organizations (PPOs)* allow patients to seek health care services from a preauthorized list of providers.
- *Point of service (POS)* plans enable participants to choose from approved or "network" providers but also to go "out of network," though usually with higher co-pays and deductibles, if they choose.

Medicaid is a program funded jointly by the federal and state governments to provide health insurance to people with limited incomes who also meet other eligibility criteria.

Medicare is a federal program that provides health insurance to people older than 65 and to those who are disabled and meet eligibility requirements.

State Children's Health Insurance Program (CHIP) is a joint federal and state program that provides health insurance for uninsured children. Eligibility criteria vary depending on state of residence.

Issues of Concern in Neurofibromatosis

Reading through insurance policies may be daunting, yet the effort is worth it. When choosing health insurance coverage, people with neurofibromatosis and their families should be concerned especially with the following issues.[1]

Authorization: The plan may require that specified medical services be authorized before the insurance plan will cover them. If such approval is required, determine who needs to provide it before seeking the services.

Authorized and unauthorized benefits: Sometimes the easiest way to determine what is covered in a given policy is to read the section on "unauthorized" or "excluded" services. Most medical tests and services needed by people with neurofibromatosis are covered in standard plans, but it pays to make sure ahead of time. Sometimes clauses that exclude plastic surgery for cosmetic reasons are used to deny benefits for the removal of dermal neurofibromas in neurofibromatosis 1 (NF1). If this situation arises or is anticipated, contact the surgeon who recommends a procedure. He or she can usually provide a billing code to categorize the operation as medically necessary.

Co-pays or co-insurance: Some plans require that a participant pay a specified amount per office visit or contribute a percentage of the cost of a medical test or hospital stay.

Deductible: Some plans require that participants pay a fixed number of dollars per year to cover medical expenses before the plan begins to cover services.

Drug formulary: If the plan provides coverage for prescription drugs, it may limit coverage to those medications on its approved formulary list. Ask for the formulary list to determine whether a needed medication is covered.

Lifetime caps: Some plans specify a maximum dollar amount of benefits available to a plan participant over the course of a lifetime, or for a noted condition. It pays to read the fine print ahead of time rather than find out in the midst of receiving medical treatment.

Preexisting condition clause: Some plans impose a waiting period before covering services for a preexisting condition such as neurofibromas, schwannomas, scoliosis, and other manifestations of neurofibromatosis. These clauses apply only to new participants. When people with neurofibromatosis switch jobs or health care providers, this clause can become an issue. It may require that participants wait 6 months, a year, or longer, depending on the plan, before receiving coverage or reimbursement for designated medical services. Before changing jobs or health insurers, it is important to consider whether doing without services for a specified period, or paying for them directly, is an option.

Provider network: If the plan restricts care to an authorized list of providers, check to determine whether your physicians are on the list. If not, out-of-network co-pays and other costs may apply. It may be possible to add the physician to the authorized list, but this requires the physician to contact the insurance plan administrator.

Specialists: Some plans restrict access to specialists by requiring preauthorization or by limiting the type of specialty services covered. Because people with neurofibromatosis often need to consult with and be treated by specialists, it pays to read this section of the plan carefully.

COBRA

The Consolidated Omnibus Budget Reconciliation Act of 1985 (COBRA) is a federal law that mandates conversion of an employer-sponsored group health insurance plan to a private plan for eligible individuals who terminate their jobs (by quitting, or being laid off or fired) or who become disabled and unable to continue working. COBRA applies only to companies with 20 or more employees, and employees who want to continue insurance coverage must elect to do so within 60 days of terminating employment. The former employee assumes responsibility for paying the monthly health insurance premium at the group rate plus a small administrative charge. COBRA generally allows such coverage for 18 months following job termination as long as the employee pays the monthly premium on time. COBRA can provide a health insurance bridge for people with neurofibromatosis who have lost their jobs or are waiting to become eligible for coverage by a new employer.

Appealing a Health Insurance Company's Decision

When a health insurance company declines to pay for a medical service or test, the insured individual can appeal the decision. The exact appeals procedure used depends on the health insurance company, but following a few general guidelines may make the process easier.

Determine the proper procedure: Each health insurance company has its own appeals process. Read the health insurance policy to learn how to initiate an appeal, or contact an employer's plan administrator. Another option is to call the health insurer's customer service line and ask for the proper forms.

Submit the appeal in writing: It is always best to document and submit the issue in writing, even if you talk by phone with a customer service representative. Clearly identify which medical procedure has been denied and why you believe it should be covered. A letter from your physician documenting your claim helps to bolster the appeal.

Establish timeframes for follow-up: When communicating with health insurance company representatives, always ask about how the appeal will be heard and when a decision will be made. Follow up to ensure that the appeal moves along.

Have a plan B: If the appeal is denied and you still think you have a case, one alternative is to contact an attorney for advice. Another is to contact the state government department that regulates health insurance companies (usually a department of health or business regulation). Another option is to contact the Patient Advocate Foundation, a national nonprofit organization that assists people on issues related to health insurance coverage. (Call 800–532–5274 or visit the Web site at www.patientadvocate.org.)

◆ Life Insurance

Some employers provide life insurance policies for employees. People with neurofibromatosis who are unable to obtain employer-sponsored life insurance can apply for individual policies. Although the rules vary by state and insurance company, such applications usually require a physical examination and release of medical records. Some people with neurofibromatosis have been denied individual life insurance policies because of concerns about serious medical complications that may result in premature death. This is a tough issue to handle because life insurance companies are under no obligation to insure everyone who applies and tend to make conservative decisions in the interest of reducing financial liability. One option is to speak with your physician before applying for life insurance so that any release of medical records is accompanied by information that places the complications of neurofibromatosis in context. Another option is to apply to another life insurance company, which may have different underwriting requirements. If several life insurance companies turn you down, consider applying to a company that specializes in high-risk policies. Names of such companies are available through insurance brokers.

◆ Disability Insurance

People with neurofibromatosis may become temporarily or permanently disabled and unable to work because of medical complications caused by their condition or its treatment. Sometimes people who have undergone surgery need time to recover physically before returning to work. Others may lose vision, hearing, or mobility. Chronic severe pain can also become disabling.

People who are employed and become temporarily unable to work are eligible to collect temporary disability insurance (TDI) from the state government. TDI deductions are included in the normal payroll deductions from an employee's paycheck. Eligibility criteria and benefits vary by state, so check with the state Department of Labor, or similar department, for details.

If the disability is expected to last for more than 12 months, individuals are eligible for federal disability payments made by the Social Security Administration (SSA). Two programs are available through SSA. Social Security Disability Insurance (SSDI) provides income for disabled people who were previously employed in jobs covered by Social Security. Benefits under SSDI are determined by how much a person earned while working. Supplemental Security Insurance (SSI) is a similar program for people who are age 65 and older, blind, or disabled and have a low income and are without financial assets. Benefits under SSI vary by state, depending on whether and how much the state supplements federal benefits.

The application process for SSDI and SSI can be lengthy and daunting, but it is possible for people with neurofibromatosis to receive benefits. Much of the advice that follows was provided by someone with NF1 who successfully obtained benefits and wrote a book full of helpful advice about how others could do so.[2] The first step is to contact a local SSA office (every state has at least one) or go online at www.ssa.gov to obtain an application. Be forewarned that the application is long and requires medical history and supporting materials from physicians. It is best to apply for benefits as soon as it becomes clear that the disability may last at least 12 months because the review process itself takes at least 4 months. Also keep in mind that you are not eligible to collect benefits until you are disabled for 5 consecutive months. (To use an example: If Jane Doe becomes disabled on February 1 and applies for benefits immediately, she will not learn of SSA's decision about whether she is eligible for benefits until May 1. Even if eligible, she will not be able to receive benefits until June 1.)

To make the application process easier:

- *Provide detailed answers:* The SSA application is long and may seem complicated because you need to supply dates and details from your medical records. Remember that the more details you provide, the better. Include supporting information such as copies of bills and medical records if appropriate.
- *Keep a copy of the application:* This may seem obvious, but many people forget. A copy of the submitted application comes in handy should you need to contact SSA or are asked a question about something you wrote down.
- *Follow up:* Call or e-mail SSA after submitting your application to make sure it was received and ask when a decision will be made. (The normal review process is 120 days.) You can also send the application via certified mail, return receipt requested, so that you have a record of having sent it. If you do not receive a letter from SSA detailing the decision by the appointed date, call to make sure the application has not been lost or misplaced.

Many people are turned down the first time they apply for SSA benefits, but the decision can be appealed. Some people appeal more than one time. To ensure that an appeal goes smoothly, take the following steps:

- *Keep the denial letter:* The SSA is obligated to explain in writing why an application is turned down. The denial letter contains valuable information, such as why you were turned down and what health care providers and hospitals were listed in your application. Sometimes the list is incomplete, indicating that the SSA administrator did not review all of the information originally included in the application. The letter should also indicate whom to contact at the SSA to request an appeal.
- *Use the proper procedure:* People have 60 days to appeal a denial from SSA. Use the proper form, known as a "request for reconsideration," which can be obtained from any SSA office.

- *Consider hiring a disability lawyer:* Some people prefer to hire an attorney to fight for benefits. Hire an attorney with experience in disability cases. If cost is an issue, look for an attorney who works on a contingency basis (paid only if benefits are awarded).
- *Contact your representative:* Don't be afraid to contact your U.S. senator or congressman for help in obtaining SSA benefits. Each federal representative has a state or district office. Simply call the local congressional office, ask for constituent relations, and explain that you are applying for SSI or SSDI benefits and having difficulty obtaining them. You should be connected with whoever handles liaison with SSA for the congressional office.

◆ Employment Discrimination

People with neurofibromatosis and their loved ones sometimes encounter discrimination in employment. Some people have been denied a job or promotion they are qualified for because of an employer's misguided concerns that the condition is contagious or might alienate customers. Other people have been fired or demoted because they took too much sick leave. Technically, such behavior is illegal, but it happens.

Two federal laws prohibit discrimination due to illness or a genetic condition such as neurofibromatosis. The Americans with Disabilities Act of 1990 (ADA) prohibits discrimination on the basis of a physical or mental impairment and requires that employers with more than 15 employees provide "reasonable" accommodations for eligible employees. Examples of reasonable accommodations include modifications in the work environment to make it accessible or flexible scheduling to accommodate medical appointments. The ADA also prohibits employers from asking someone about a medical condition during a job interview or refusing to hire someone out of concern that the employee or his family will incur big medical expenses. The Family and Medical Leave Act of 1993 enables employees who have worked for the same employer for 12 months or longer to take an unpaid 12-week leave for serious medical reasons. This leave can be taken if the employee himself needs care or if a family member needs care. After the leave ends, the employee must resume the original job or be assigned one that is similar in terms of pay and benefits.

For further information about these laws, or to file a charge of discrimination, contact the federal Equal Employment Opportunity Commission, your state Human Rights Commission, or the federal or state Department of Labor. Another option is to consult with an attorney familiar with employment law.

◆ Physical Limitations

Most people with neurofibromatosis do not have to limit their activities in any way, nor are they more prone to injury than others. Some people, however, may be faced with complications that limit mobility and function temporarily and even permanently. People with NF1 who have scoliosis or bone abnormalities, for instance, may need temporary bracing and/or physical therapy. People with NF2 who have vestibular schwannomas may benefit from balance exercises whether or not they have surgery. Anyone with neurofibromatosis-related pain may try to avoid triggering more by altering posture or movements, but in the long run this may cause a different pain elsewhere. Severe physical limitations and pain can alter the ability to work, and to participate in sports or exercise, hobbies, social activities, and home maintenance.

Pain management strategies are discussed below. These may be used in conjunction with physical and/or occupational therapy, depending on the individual's condition. Although there is a lot of overlap between the two professions, physical therapists tend to focus on the entire body, whereas occupational therapists focus more on the upper extremities. Both teach exercises to strengthen muscles and recommend assistive devices such as splints and canes to ease pressure on sore areas of the body.

◆ Pain Management

The word *pain* is derived from the Latin term for penalty or punishment. Certainly anyone with neurofibromatosis who has experienced it can attest that sometimes this is exactly how severe pain feels. There is no easy solution to the medical perplexities of pain, but there are multiple therapeutic options that may provide full or partial relief.[3,4]

Pain is usually classified in one of three ways. Transient pain hurts, but passes within hours. This type of pain occurs when someone with NF1 bumps a neurofibroma, or when anyone bangs a knee or cuts a finger. Tension headaches and some migraines fall into this category. Acute pain is more severe and lasts longer than transient pain, although it does eventually recede. People with neurofibromatosis may experience acute pain while recovering from surgery, having a migraine, or as a result of spinal tumors that compress nerve roots. Chronic pain persists far longer than acute pain and is the toughest form of pain to treat. People with schwannomatosis and those with NF1 and NF2 who have inoperable tumors that are pressing on nerves may also experience chronic pain.

Diagnosis

The first step in evaluating pain is to try to find the cause. Symptoms are of primary importance in this regard. No medical test or imaging device can gauge the intensity of pain, although they may help pinpoint the cause of it. Physicians rely on the patient's description of where the pain is located, how long it lasts, and what it feels like. Use words like *dull* or *sharp, constant* or *transient, aching* or *burning* to describe pain; this helps the physician to zero in on a potential cause. The physician may order x-rays, magnetic resonance imaging (MRI) scans, or other medical tests to locate tumors or other abnormalities. Although it is frustrating for patient and physician alike, it is not always possible to determine immediately what is causing the pain.

It is vitally important to consider malignant peripheral nerve sheath tumors (MPNSTs) as a possible cause of chronic pain in people with NF1. As mentioned in Chapter 6, a delay in diagnosing an MPNST can mean the difference between life and death. For that reason, even if pain treatment is initiated, it is wise to arrange follow-up testing until an MPNST can be ruled out.

Treatment

Pain relief in neurofibromatosis depends on the cause. Sometimes the best way to relieve pain caused by a tumor pressing on a nerve is to remove the tumor. If complete excision is not possible, a partial removal that reduces the size of the tumor may provide some relief. When tumors are inoperable or—as is common in neurofibromatosis—the cause of pain is unknown, medications and other interventions may provide some relief.

Physicians usually begin with conservative treatments first and then try more aggressive options if these initial strategies do not work. Many medications have side effects, so be sure to check with a physician and/or pharmacist before choosing one. Anecdotal information from friends or family members is not always helpful, for individuals metabolize drugs in different ways. What works for your friend with neurofibromatosis may not work for you. It is also important to understand that neuropathic pain, which is caused by damage to a nerve, may not respond to standard pain medications and may require treatment with drugs normally used for other conditions such as epilepsy.

People with neurofibromatosis who are unable to find pain relief through the methods described below may want to consider seeking a consultation with a pain specialist or at a specialized pain clinic. This is a relatively new field of medicine with specialists who may be aware of options other physicians do not yet know about.

Over-the-counter pain relievers are usually the first medications recommended if the pain is mild to moderate in severity. These include aspirin, acetaminophen (brand names include *Anacin* and *Tylenol*), and nonsteroidal anti-inflammatory drugs (NSAIDs) such as ibuprofen (*Advil, Motrin IB,* etc.), ketoprofen *(Actron, Orudis KT),* and naproxen sodium *(Aleve).* Some medications contain a mixture of ingredients. For instance, one over-the-counter medication, *Excedrin Migraine,* combines aspirin, acetaminophen, and caffeine. Over-the-counter medications must be paid out-of-pocket, because health insurers do not cover them.

Prescription pain relievers may be necessary for moderate to severe pain. These medications must be ordered by a physician and are usually obtained at pharmacies. Examples include NSAIDs such as diclofenac sodium *(Voltaren),* ibuprofen *(Motrin),* ketoprofen *(Orudis, Oruvail),* nabumetone *(Relafen),* and naproxen *(Naprosyn).* Such NSAIDs work by blocking two enzymes involved in the transmission of pain signals to the brain, known as Cox-1 and Cox-2. Medications known as Cox-2 inhibitors block only the second enzyme and cause fewer gastrointestinal reactions than NSAIDs. Cox-2 inhibitors include celecoxib *(Celebrex)* and others in development. Drugs intended specifically for migraine headaches include ergotamine *(Ergomar, Ergostat),* naratriptan *(Amerge),* rizatriptan *(Maxalt),* zolmitriptan *(Zomig),* and sumatriptan *(Imitrex).* Some health insurers do provide partial or complete reimbursement for prescription drugs, although choice of drug may be restricted.

Opioid medications, also known as narcotics, are prescription medicines reserved for severe or recalcitrant pain. Opioids tend to be sedating, causing drowsiness, and they can become addictive. As a result, physicians may be reluctant to prescribe them. Even given the risks, however, opioids may be a viable option for people with neurofibromatosis who are experiencing severe pain that has not responded to other treatments. Anyone taking opioids should be monitored regularly; side effects vary and doses must be calibrated carefully. Opioids include codeine, propoxyphene *(Darvon, Darvocet),* oxycodone *(Percodan, Percocet),* oxycodone HCI controlled-release tablets *(OxyContin),* morphine *(MS Contin, Kadian,* etc.), hydromorphone *(Dilaudid),* and fentanyl *(Duragesic patch).*

Antidepressants are sometimes prescribed in low dosages for pain caused by nerve damage, whether or not the patient has depression. They also improve sleep for some people with chronic pain. These medications work by increasing levels of serotonin and norepinephrine, two neurotransmitters that are involved in both mood and the transmission of pain signals. The antidepressants that appear to be most effective in treating nerve pain are the older or tricyclic antidepressants (named for their three-ring molecular shape). These include amitriptyline *(Elavil),* nortriptyline *(Aventyl, Pamelor),* and imipramine *(Tofranil, Janimine).*

Anticonvulsants provide another option in treating neuropathic pain. These medications, normally used in treating epilepsy and other types of seizures, block aberrant nerve cell signaling that may be involved in producing the sensation of pain. Anticonvulsants used to treat nerve pain include carbamazepine *(Tegretol),* clonazepam *(Klonopin),* gabapentin *(Neurontin),* phenytoin *(Dilantin),* and valproic acid *(Depakene).*

Cardiac medications may be prescribed for pain related to neurofibromatosis. Antiarrhythmic medications, which are usually used to correct an irregular heartbeat, can treat nerve pain. These include mexiletine *(Mexitil)* and clonidine *(Catapres).* High blood pressure medications may be effective in preventing a migraine headache or easing its symptoms. Examples include beta-blockers such as propranolol *(Inderal)* and calcium-channel blockers *(Cardizem, Procardia).*

Nerve blocks are injections to block signals generated by a specific[1] nerve. These are available for short- and long-term relief of pain in some cases. Patient-controlled analgesia delivers medication through an intravenous line from an external pump that the patient can activate as needed. Similar implantable pumps may provide an option for people whose pain has not responded to other strategies.

◆ The Personal Perspective

Nancy B: "I have worried about insurance, primarily when I've changed jobs. In one job, the insurance plan wouldn't cover any preexisting conditions for a year. So I took the chance that nothing would happen, and it didn't. But during the few times when I have seen doctors about NF-related symptoms, I haven't had any trouble with insurance."

Porter C.: "Some people with neurofibromatosis have no pain. I have. It hurts to be hugged—that is, a bear hug. Gentle hugs are okay. Sometimes the pain is sharp, like being stuck with an ice pick being wiggled around. Sometimes it's pressure pain.

"My back is impossible for me to get clean. Twice a week, someone comes to work on it with a soft toothbrush. I wear soft clothing and have to be careful trying on clothes so that I don't get anything bloody."

Kellie C.: "The people at the NF Foundation have been supportive. I think that has helped. They told us that they'd be there to support us, whatever happened."

Diane D.: "I kept records of everything, and at first I carried everything to each appointment. I had a great big notebook, and we'd review it during office visits. Now I just take the latest report. I still keep everything on file at home. I'm now up to three notebooks. I have separate ones for school records and meetings.

"I work 4 full days a week. I often work through lunch so that I can fit in all Julie's appointments. I meet regularly with school officials twice a week, and then with the psychologist and all the doctors. It can be challenging."

Dolores G.: "Susan was an exception as far as pain went. Most people with NF1 do not have as much pain as she did even early on. Of course if you bump a neurofibroma, you'd have pain. But if you have internal neurofibromas and they're growing, you might have pain. So most of her pain was from internal tumors.

"Toward the end, she was on a lot of drugs to control the pain. She took morphine and a lot of OxyContin in the last two years of her life. Her pain doctor was very good and stuck his neck out for her. He was investigated a few times because he prescribed her so much OxyContin. But that was the only thing that would help her pain. She was in excruciating pain from the internal tumors."

Marcy H.: "The pain of schwannomatosis is off the chart. If you don't go through it, you don't know how bad it is. It's like living with knives in me. I can't stand it. I take Neurontin for pain. The maximum dose is 6000 mg a day, and although I'm only 89 pounds, that's often what I'm taking.

Table 14–1   Sample Patient Information Tracking Sheet

Name:
Date of birth:
Sex:
Mother's name:
Father's name:
Primary care physician (name, address, phone number):
Eye doctor (name, address, phone number):
Other medical providers (names, addresses, phone numbers):

Adapted from Patient Information Sheet, Understanding NF1, www.understandingnf1.org, with permission of the University of Alabama at Birmingham Department of Genetics.

Table 14–2   Sample Medical Visit Tracking Sheet

Date of visit:

Where visit occurred:

Reason for visit:

Follow-up appointment:

Materials received (i.e., tests, x-rays):

Nurses and specialties of medical professionals seen:

Notes:

Adapted from Visit Summaries, Understanding NF1, www.understandingnf1.org, with permission of the University of Alabama at Birmingham Department of Genetics.

Table 14–3   Sample Medical Visit Worksheet

Before the appointment

Keep notes of topics you would like to discuss with your doctor.
• Information and questions about NF, changes you have noticed, etc.

Collect things to take to the appointment.
• Test results, photographs, documents.

At the appointment

Take notes about information you receive from the medical professionals and note any tests that were performed.

After the appointment

List the things to do as a result of the appointment.
• Schedule consultation with another medical professional.
• Arrange for a test or call for test results.
• Send information to medical provider.
• Receive information from medical provider.

Adapted from Visit Worksheet, Understanding NF1, www.understandingnf1.org, with permission of the University of Alabama at Birmingham Department of Genetics.

"Biofeedback has worked for me. I go through a series of relaxation exercises, working from my head to my toes. I become so relaxed that I actually am alleviating much of the pain. With lots of practice, I've been able to use biofeedback without anesthesia during surgery."

Martha L.: "I don't know sign language, and in some ways refuse to learn it. I know, I'm stubborn, but I feel if I stop using the abilities I have to carry on a normal conversation with someone, then NF has won. I do have a little hearing left, and I make sure I can see the person's mouth when I am talking with them. I need to be able to communicate with people in both my professional and private lives, and for the sake of my own sanity."

References

1. Psychosocial Aspects of the Neurofibromatoses: Impact on the Individual, Impact on the Family. Jane Novak Pugh Conference Series, vol. 3. New York: National Neurofibromatosis Foundation; 1992

2. Silesky S. The Secrets to Getting Disability Benefits: How to Survive Financially and Emotionally When Injury or Illness Threatens Your Livelihood. Bellevue, WA: Ki Health Inc., Education and Development Services Division; 2002

3. Pain. Hope Through Research. National Institute of Neurological Disorders and Stroke Web site. Available at: http://www.ninds.nih.gov/health_and_medical/pubs/pain.htm.

4. Wehrwein P. What to Do About Pain. Boston, MA: Harvard Health Publications; 2000

15

Research About Neurofibromatosis

Although the past decade has yielded many new insights into the genetic and molecular abnormalities that cause neurofibromatosis, many questions remain about how its manifestations develop and how to manage them. Most disturbing to patients and families is the fact that there is currently no way to prevent these disorders or cure them. At the same time, physicians and families are hopeful that as more is learned about neurofibromatosis, effective treatments will be found. Scientific research is essential for achieving this goal.

Basic research is directed at understanding the inherent biological processes of disorders. Many of the molecular-genetic insights into neurofibromatosis detailed in Chapter 3 resulted from basic research in the laboratories. Current research is directed at better understanding the function of the *NF1* and *NF2* genes, identifying the mechanisms responsible for schwannomatosis, and identifying molecular targets that could serve as the basis of therapy. The development of animal models to study these and other research questions in vivo (in a living body), as well as in the laboratory, is essential.

Clinical research tests new treatments and evaluates the timing and type of interventions used, to determine which treatments are optimal. The management recommendations detailed in this book are based on the outcome of clinical research. Clinical research now underway is aimed at better determining optimal timing of therapies for certain tumors, the natural history of neurofibromatosis, and quality-of-life issues.

◆ Clinical Trials

People with neurofibromatosis and family members who are eager to support clinical research can do so by enrolling in clinical trials, which evaluate and compare the effectiveness of potential therapies. Clinical trials provide the critical link between basic laboratory research and improved treatments. Typically these trials are conducted in stages over several years. The preclinical phase refers to tests in the laboratory and in animal models. If a therapy looks promising, research advances to a phase one trial, the first to occur in people. Phase one trials involve a relatively small number of people who have not responded to other therapies for their distinct medical condition. The goal is to determine whether a new medication or treatment is safe. Phase two trials then determine whether the treatment is effective. Typically the new treatment is compared with an existing therapy or to a placebo, a harmless but ineffectual medication or other treatment that should have no therapeutic effect. Assuming the new treatment is safe and effective, it moves into the final phase of testing known as a phase three trial. This phase usually involves many people nationwide. The goal is to determine whether a new treatment is more effective than current therapies and what types of benefits and side effects it offers.

Conducting clinical research that moves a discovery from "bench to bedside" can take an estimated 12 to 20 years. Most promising agents discovered in laboratories do not make it onto drugstore shelves. This can be disappointing for both researchers and patients. In the case of NF1, for instance, early laboratory studies indicated that it might be possible to inhibit Ras, one of the molecules that contribute to neurofibroma growth. So far, clinical studies of a few Ras-inhibiting agents in people have not lived up to expectations. On the other hand, clinical trials have helped to determine which surgical techniques are most effective for managing tumors associated with neurofibromatosis.

◆ Participating in a Clinical Trial

People who want to participate in clinical trials must meet certain conditions known as enrollment criteria. These vary depending on the issue under study. Participants must also be willing to have periodic medical follow-up visits. Benefits of participation include the opportunity to increase knowledge about neurofibromatosis and options for therapy and in some cases the chance to gain early access to a treatment that may be better than traditional options. Any study involves risks that can range from minimal (pain when having blood drawn) to more serious concerns (a new treatment may offer no benefit over standard therapy, or the true risks of treatment may not yet be known).

Participation in a clinical trial is voluntary and can take place only after someone has provided informed consent. Before signing an informed consent form, a person must be fully informed about the purpose of the study, its procedures, risks, and potential benefits. The informed consent form should include details about the study, risks and benefits, whom to contact with questions, and how to withdraw from the study at any time. If any aspect of the study or the wording of an informed consent form is not clear and fully understood, ask questions. The researchers running the study understand that participants may not be medical professionals, and they should be prepared to explain everything in plain language.

In many clinical trials, participation is free of charge. The grant funding a research study generally covers the costs of medications, study-related medical visits, and laboratory tests. At other times, the institution sponsoring the study may cover such costs. It is wise to ask about cost of participation ahead of time, however. Health insurance plans rarely cover the costs of experimental therapies and are unlikely to pay for participation in a clinical trial.

The NF Foundation maintains an ongoing list of clinical trials open to participants with neurofibromatosis. For more information, visit the NF Foundation Web site: www.nf.org. As always, check with a physician or other trusted health care provider before making a final decision about participating.

◆ An Exciting Time in Neurofibromatosis Research

Research into neurofibromatosis operates on the cutting edge of modern science. Each year, the NF Foundation sponsors two major medical symposia. The NNFF International Consortium for the Molecular Biology of NF1 and NF2 usually meets in the spring. The Annual NF Symposium is held during the annual meeting of the American Society for Human Genetics. Both forums enable brilliant scientists who are leaders in their fields to share the latest discoveries in areas as diverse as molecular biology, biochemistry, gene function, development of animal models, and new treatment strategies. These meetings also attract distinguished researchers from outside the field whose discoveries and knowledge may provide insight into neurofibromatosis. In addition, the NF Foundation funds young investigator grants to encourage promising scientists at the start of their careers and fosters numerous informal collaborations throughout the year. The challenges of neurofibromatosis are many, but the future has never looked brighter, thanks in large part to the progress and the promise of scientific discovery.

Appendix

◆ **The National Neurofibromatosis Foundation, Inc.**

The National Neurofibromatosis Foundation, Inc., a nonprofit organization founded in 1978, is dedicated to serving the needs of people with neurofibromatosis and their families. Towards that end, the NF Foundation supports research into the causes and treatment of neurofibromatosis, provides information about these disorders, and sponsors a broad range of outreach efforts. A brief sampling of programs is listed below. To learn more, call 800-323-7938 or visit the NF Foundation Web site: www.nf.org.

Research

The Research Advisory Board and Clinical Care Advisory Board include renowned physicians and scientists who are experts about neurofibromatosis and schwannomatosis. With guidance from these boards, the NF Foundation sponsors research studies and establishes standards of excellence for clinical care. As an aid to patients, the NF Foundation also maintains a list of studies and clinical trials that are seeking participants.

Information and Support

To better educate patients, families, and the public, the NF Foundation sponsors symposia, publishes books, brochures, newsletters and educational materials, and maintains an active Web site. Information in Spanish is available on the Web site and in printed form upon request.

To aid patients in finding a doctor, the NF Foundation maintains a list of specialty clinics in the United States and around the world. Any center listed must meet the Foundation's criteria. For individuals who are interested in local activities and support, a list of state chapters and international affiliates is available, as well as an online Bulletin Board and Chat Room accessed by visiting the NF Foundation's Web site: www.nf.org.

Glossary

ADD: Attention deficit disorder, characterized by inability to focus and pay attention.

ADHD: Attention deficit hyperactivity disorder, which combines inability to focus with hyperactivity and inability to sit still.

Angiogram: An X-ray or MRI image of blood vessels taken after a dye has been injected into them.

Astrocytoma: A brain tumor that develops from astrocytes, star-shaped glial cells. Always malignant but may be low-grade.

Audiogram: Test of hearing ability.

Autosomal dominant: A pattern of inheritance in which only one gene in a pair needs to be altered to cause a trait or disorder. A person born with such a gene has a 50% chance of passing it on to any of his or her children. NF1 and NF2 are both autosomal dominant disorders.

Axon: An extension from a neuron that enables it to send signals to other neurons.

BAER (Brainstem auditory evoked responses): Test of the brain pathway involved in hearing.

Benign tumor: An abnormal growth that does not spread to or invade surrounding tissues. Depending on location, may cause symptoms such as pain and loss of function and even may result in death if the tumor interferes with a vital function like breathing.

Bilateral: Affecting or present on both sides of the body, such as both ears.

Biopsy: Surgical removal of tissue for analysis to aid diagnosis.

Café-au-lait spots: Areas that are darker in color than surrounding skin, variable in shape and size, present on people with NF1.

Cancer: An abnormal and uncontrolled growth of cells that can spread to and invade other tissues. Most tumors that occur in neurofibromatosis are not cancerous.

Cataract: A clouding of the eye lens that can cause vision loss; the type known as juvenile posterior subcapsular lenticular opacity may occur in NF2.

Central nervous system: Brain and spinal cord.

Chemotherapy: Treatment of malignant tumors and other types of aberrant cell growth with chemical agents.

Chromosomes: Structures located in the cell nucleus that contain genes determining hereditary characteristics. Each person has 23 pairs of chromosomes.

Congenital: Present at birth.

Cranial: Related to the skull.

CT scan: Computerized tomography, an imaging technique that uses a computer to assemble a series of X-rays taken at different angles to produce an image.

Discrete neurofibroma: A well-defined tumor that originates from a single site. Discrete neurofibromas are visible when they are on or near the skin.

DNA: Deoxyribonucleic acid, the chemical substance that constitutes genes.

Dominant: Only one gene in a pair needs to be altered in order to express a trait or disorder.

Dysplasia: Abnormal growth or development in a bone or tissue anywhere in the body.

Ependymoma: Tumor that develops from cells lining the cavities of the brain and spinal cord.

Epilepsy: A disorder caused by electrical abnormality in the brain that can manifest as disturbances in movement and consciousness.

Exon: The coding region of a gene.

Expessivity: Degree to which a genetic trait is manifested.

Familial neurofibromatosis: Inherited from a parent who has the disorder.

Gene: The basic unit of heredity, made up of strands of DNA. Genes, like chromosomes, exist in pairs.

Genetic testing: Analysis of a blood or tissue sample to determine whether someone has a particular genetic mutation.

Genotype/phenotype correlation: The association between a gene and its physical manifestations.

Glial cells: Specialized cells in the nervous system that support the functioning of neurons.

Glioma: A type of brain tumor that arises from glial cells that support nerve cells.

Haploinsufficiency: A situation in which normal levels of a protein cannot be produced in a cell, which may result in manifestations of a disorder.

Hormone: Chemical substance secreted by a gland, which performs a precise function in the body.

Hydrocephalus: Increased spinal fluid pressure within the ventricles of the brain.

Hypertension: High blood pressure.

Hypertrophy: Increase in the size of a part of the body.

Hypothalamus: Part of the brain responsible for control of hormone secretion, appetite, and other "automatic" functions.

Kyphosis: A hump in the upper portion of the spine. Sometimes seen in conjunction with lateral scoliosis in individuals with NF1.

Learning disability: A neurological disorder that affects the brain's ability to receive, process, store, and respond to information. Describes a group of disorders. Learning disabilities can hinder a person's ability to listen, read, write, spell, speak, or do math calculations, even though he or she has average or above average intelligence.

Lisch nodules: Small clumps of pigment on the iris of the eye that do not interfere with vision. They are seen in people with NF1.

Macrocephaly: A head that is larger than normal in circumference. Does not cause medical complications.

MRI: The abbreviation for magnetic resonance imaging, a diagnostic technique that uses a powerful magnet and computers to provide images of organs and tissue inside the body. MRI is particularly useful in visualizing the brain.

Malignant peripheral nerve sheath tumor: A malignant tumor that usually originates in a plexiform neurofibroma.

Malignant tumor: An abnormal growth capable of invading other tissues and spreading to other areas of the body. Also known as cancer. Must be treated or death will result.

Meningioma: A benign tumor of the covering of the brain and spinal cord.

Merlin: Protein product of the NF2 gene. Also known as schwannomin.

Mitogenic signals: Signals that induce a cell to divide into two identical cells.

Mosaic neurofibromatosis: A variation of neurofibromatosis in which features associated with the disorder develop only in one part of the body. Thought to be the result of a gene mutation that occurs after conception and exists in only some cells in the body.

MPNST: The common abbreviation for malignant peripheral nerve sheath tumors.

Mutation: A permanent, transmissible change in genetic material, usually in a single gene.

Myelin: The substance that forms a covering that insulates nerves and improves the transmission of signals from one nerve to the next.

Neural crest: An embryonic structure that produces many of the cell types that, in neurofibromatosis, deviate from their proper course. Includes nerve sheath cells.

Neuron: The basic functional and anatomical cell in the nervous system that specializes in communication.

Neurofibroma: A benign tumor that develops in the myelin sheath that surrounds peripheral nerves and contains multiple cell types. Most common tumor seen in NF1.

Neurofibromatosis: The common term for three types of genetic disorders (NF1, NF2, and schwannomatosis) which all cause the development of benign tumors in the myelin sheath that surrounds nerves.

Neurofibromin: Protein product of the NF1 gene.

NF1: The most common form of neurofibromatosis, characterized by developmental changes in the nervous system, skin, bones, and other tissues. Distinguishing manifestations include multiple café-au-lait spots and neurofibromas.

NF2: A form of neurofibromatosis whose distinguishing characteristic is the growth of vestibular schwannomas.

Optic glioma: A tumor that develops on the optic nerve, which transmits visual information from the eye to the brain. This tumor sometimes develops in people with NF1.

Palpation: A method of diagnosis that involves touching or applying pressure to an area of the body.

Papilledema: Swelling of the optic nerve.

Pathogenesis: The process by which a disorder originates and progresses.

Peripheral nervous system: Nerves that extend to the extremities and parts of the body away from the brain and spinal cord.

Pheochromocytoma: An adrenal gland tumor.

Plexiform neurofibroma: A diffuse type of neurofibroma that grows along an entire nerve shaft or envelops multiple nerves and sometimes occurs in people with NF1.

Post-zygotic mutation: A change in a gene that occurs sometime after conception.

Precocious puberty: Abnormally early onset of puberty. Sometimes occurs in NF1.

Proptosis: A condition in which the eyes push outward.

Pseudarthrosis: A false joint that sometimes develops when a fracture in a long bone does not heal in a person with NF1.

Ras: A protein that initiates cell division that is regulated, in part, by the NF1 gene.

Recessive: Both members of a pair of genes need to be altered in order to have expression of the trait or disorder.

RNA: Ribonucleic acid, which helps to decode the genetic instructions contained in DNA.

Schwann cell: The cell which forms the myelin that surrounds and protects peripheral nerves.

Schwannoma: A benign tumor that develops from Schwann cells. Seen in people with NF2 and schwannomatosis.

Schwannomatosis: The most recently recognized form of neurofibromatosis, characterized by growth of multiple schwannomas anywhere except on the vestibular nerve.

Schwannomin: The protein product of the NF2 gene. Also known as merlin.

Scoliosis: A lateral (sideways) curvature of the spine, which occurs earlier in people with NF1 than in the general population.

Segmental neurofibromatosis: See mosaic neurofibromatosis.

Seizure: Uncontrolled electrical activity in the brain; can cause aberrant movement or loss of consciousness. If seizures recur, epilepsy may be diagnosed.

Signaling pathway: A sequence of biochemical events that is triggered by the activation of a particular gene.

Skin-fold freckling: A cluster of small pigmented spots that appear in areas where skin meets skin (such as the armpit or groin) in people with NF1.

Slit lamp: Device used by ophthalmologists to examine structures at the front of the eyes. Needed for proper examination for Lisch nodules.

Sphenoid: Skull bone that forms a portion of the back of the eye socket. Sometimes abnormal in people with NF1.

Spontaneous mutation: A change in a gene that occurs by chance rather than as a result of an external factor. Such changes may account for non-inherited cases of neurofibromatosis.

Sporadic neurofibromatosis: Occurs in an individual because of a spontaneous genetic mutation. There is no family history of the disorder.

Strabismus: Inability to focus both eyes in parallel on the same point.

Syndrome: A group of symptoms or manifestations that constitute a disorder when they occur together.

Tibia: Long bone at the front of lower leg (shin bone), sometimes bowed in people with NF1.

Tinnitus: Ringing in the ears. May be an early sign of vestibular schwannoma.

Tumor: An abnormal uncontrolled growth of cells. Tumors may be benign or malignant.

Tumor suppressor: A gene that, when functioning normally, controls cell growth and division and prevents tumors from forming.

UBO: Unidentified bright object, an area of hyperintensity on an MRI of the brain that is sometimes seen in NF1, most often in children. Significance is not known.

Unilateral: Affecting or present on one side of the body, such as one ear.

Vertebrae: Bones forming the spinal column.

Vestibular schwannoma: Benign tumor that originates in the vestibular branch of the eighth cranial nerve (which conveys sense of balance information to the brain), but often compresses the acoustic branch causing hearing loss. Defining feature of NF2.

Index

Numbers followed by "f" or "t" indicate that the entry on that page is in a figure or table.